YOUR DOCTOR HAS TOLD YOU
YOU'RE A CANDIDATE FOR
HIP OR KNEE REPLACEMENT SURGERY . . .
BUT WHAT *HASN'T* YOUR DOCTOR TOLD YOU?
NOW GET ALL OF YOUR QUESTIONS ANSWERED:

- Do I need joint replacement just because the X-rays "look bad"?

- How long should my replacement last?

- Can pain between my upper thigh and belly be caused by a hip problem?

- Is the whole knee removed in total knee replacement?

- Is it possible to be too old for a hip replacement?

- Will I be able to play tennis after my joint replacement?

- Will my joint replacement create problems for me with airport security?

- Are there warning signs before a hip dislocates?

- What's the big deal about a "revision" (redo) joint replacement?

- Can I get an MRI if I've had a joint replacement?

Don't get on the operating table until you get all the facts. With accuracy, compassion, and candor, noted expert Dr. Ronald P. Grelsamer responds to your concerns and explains . . .

WHAT YOUR DOCTOR MAY *NOT* TELL YOU
ABOUT™ HIP AND KNEE
REPLACEMENT SURGERY

ALSO BY RONALD R. GRELSAMER, M.D.:

*What Your Doctor May Not Tell You About
Knee Pain and Surgery*

WHAT YOUR DOCTOR MAY *NOT* TELL YOU ABOUT™

HIP AND KNEE REPLACEMENT SURGERY

Everything You Need to Know to Make the Right Decisions

RONALD P. GRELSAMER, M.D.
author of *What Your Doctor May Not Tell You About*™
Knee Pain and Surgery

WARNER BOOKS

NEW YORK   BOSTON

The information herein is not intended to replace the services of trained health professionals, or be a substitute for medical advice. You are advised to consult with your health care professional with regard to matters relating to your health, and in particular regarding matters that may require diagnosis or medical attention.

Warner Books
Time Warner Book Group
1271 Avenue of the Americas, New York, NY 10020
Visit our Web site at www.twbookmark.com.

Printed in the United States of America

First Printing: April 2004

10 9 8 7 6 5 4 3 2 1

Library of Congress Cataloging-in-Publication Data
Grelsamer, Ronald P.
    What your doctor may not tell you about hip and knee replacement surgery : everything you need to know to make the right decisions / Ronald P. Grelsamer.
        p. cm.
    Includes bibliographical references and index.
    ISBN 0-446-67977-1
    1. Hip Joint—Surgery—Popular works. 2. Total hip replacement—Popular works.
3. Knee—Surgery—Popular works. 4. Consumer education. I. Title.
    RD549.G74 2004
    617.5'810592—dc22   2003023911

Cover design by Diane Luger
Book design by Charles A. Sutherland

Acknowledgments

My patients first and foremost deserve my thanks for trusting me with their knees and hips. Moreover, you, my patients, have provided many of the topics covered in this book—especially the Questions and Answers.

My immediate colleagues Drs. Allan Strongwater, Jack Choueka, Jean-Pierre Farcy, Jeffrey Klein, Hershel Samuels, Frank Schwab, Vladimir Shur, and Drew Stein as well as my colleagues at the Maimonides Medical Center and the Hospital for Joint Diseases have provided constant encouragement.

Once again, the patience of my wife, Sharon, and of my children, Dominique and Marc, has been invaluable.

In my office, Lori Swanson, Carine Bristout, Michelle Roberts, Andria Cameron and John Carrique have held the fort.

Thank you to Lillian Reilly and her 8 West team.

John Aherne at Warner Books and Gareth Esersky have provided a steady hand throughout this project.

I would not be performing joint replacement surgery were it not for the teachings of my mentors Frank Stinchfield, M.D., Nas Eftekhar, M.D. and Howard Kiernan, M.D.

Finally, of course, eternal thanks to my parents for having provided me with an outstanding education.

Contents

Introduction

WHY YOU NEED THIS BOOK

You probably want more information than the average patient, more information than what your surgeon has time for in one or two consultations. And that is the key word: time. To be fully informed about every single aspect of joint replacement takes time—about the time it takes to read this book.

What's more, not everyone looks for the same information and your surgeon can't know exactly what will be of greatest interest to you. Do you really want to know about every single complication, or are you more interested in detailed explanations of the do's and don'ts after surgery? With this book in hand, you can pick and choose your particular areas of interests.

In our companion book (*What Your Doctor May* Not *Tell You About Knee Pain and Surgery,* Warner Books, 2002), I introduced the concept of the LK-SS doctor (Limited Knowledge–Suspect Scruples). When suffering from knee pain, you won't get the information you need if your doctor is lacking in knowledge or scruples. This is particularly true when it comes to so-called torn cartilage and MRIs.

The situation is different in the world of hip and knee replacements. There are fewer ways that your surgeon can trick you into thinking you need a joint replacement (we discuss that in chapter 2). To paraphrase Jagger-Richards, you may get the information you need, but not all the information you want.

In this book I cover the basics, and I also discuss aspects of joint replacement that the average patient may be less interested in—information that *you* will find intriguing and that will make you a more informed consumer.

When the doctor throws you a morsel of information that you don't completely grasp, you can come right to this book.

Meet me at the beginning of chapter 1 to discuss who really needs a hip or a knee replacement.

Part I

AN OVERVIEW

Chapter 1

❖❖❖

Who Needs a Joint Replacement? Arthritis, AVN, and Femoral Neck (Hip) Fractures

There isn't as much deception with joint replacement surgery as there is with outpatient arthroscopies (see *What Your Doctor May* Not *Tell You About Knee Pain and Surgery*, Warner Books, 2002). If your doctor has suggested a joint replacement, you are probably a reasonable candidate for the procedure. The only thing to quibble about is timing. Do you really need it now? During an arthritic flare-up, you'll agree to just about anything, including major surgery. Of course, this flare-up will quiet down, especially if it's one of the first. The unscrupulous doctor may quickly sign you up for surgery without informing you that arthritis pain typically waxes and wanes.

> It's usually not a question of whether you need a joint replacement, but rather a question of *when*? **Do you need it *now*?**

Here is a tip: If the doctor looks at your X-ray, throws a doleful look your way, and advises you of the need for a joint replacement, run out of there as fast as your arthritic legs can carry you! A good doctor treats patients, not X-rays! I'm reminded of the ninety-two-year-old man who came to see me a few years ago. He walked in and plopped his X-rays on my desk. They showed some of the worst arthritis I'd ever seen. The bones were so close together that I couldn't quite tell where one started and the other ended. I started to think about the risks associated with performing knee replacement surgery on a nonagenarian. Then he started his story: "Doc, I carry my own golf clubs, and after nine holes my knees are achy . . ." This man obviously enjoyed a great quality of life and didn't need any surgery. So much for the knee replacement. On the other hand, some people whose arthritis is barely visible on X-rays are in severe pain. So once again, I tell my students to "treat patients, not tests."

> **The word *arthritis* does not simply mean "aches and pains from old age." It has a specific definition.**

Joint replacement surgery is indicated for patients who suffer from either arthritis or avascular necrosis, also known as osteonecrosis. Certain types of hip fractures are also best treated with a hip replacement.

ARTHRITIS

Like *bursitis* and *tendinitis*, the word *arthritis* is bandied about rather loosely. But it has a specific definition: the wearing out of the articular cartilage covering the ends of a bone (figure 1.1). Look at a chicken bone. The shiny white material at the end of the bone is the articular cartilage. It is very, very smooth. Two pieces of articular cartilage gliding along each other exhibit a coefficient of friction eight times lower than two pieces of ice! When cartilage wears out, bone is exposed the way the concrete of a skating rink is laid bare by a spring-time melt. This wearing off of cartilage can be painful but, in-terestingly, not automatically so. People can live with arthritis for years without a day of pain. And then, one day, some event triggers the pain. Blunt trauma (hitting the knee against a hard object), for example, or a seem-ingly innocuous twisting injury. The triggering event isn't always obvious.

> **It's easy to think of bone as a piece of wood. It is live tissue, however, complete with a rich supply of blood vessels.**

You might come across the term *arthrosis*. For the purposes of this discussion, the term is synonymous with *arthritis*.

Not everybody with arthritis requires joint replacement surgery. A number of nonoperative treatment options exist, es-pecially for the knee. And remember: As noted above (and yes, it does warrant repeating), arthritis pain flares up and quiets down. Joint replacement surgery is not indicated until the flare-ups are lengthy and frequent.

In the next two chapters we review the surgical and non-surgical alternatives to hip and knee replacements.

OSTEONECROSIS, AKA AVASCULAR NECROSIS (AVN)

It's easy to think of bone as a piece of wood. That's because the only bone you've ever seen (presumably) is on your dinner plate. But bone is a very living tissue. It is richly supplied with

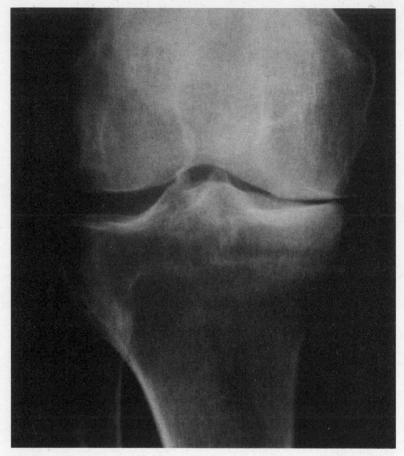

Figure 1.1 An arthritic knee. Articular cartilage is a smooth, white tissue that covers the ends of most bones. This cartilage is invisible on an X-ray and appears as an empty space. The lack of an empty space therefore indicates that the cartilage has worn down. Note how on this X-ray the bones come together.

blood vessels and it is constantly being broken down and built back up.

When blood is unable to reach part of a bone, that part literally dies. That is because bone is made of cells like any other human tissue, and when cells are deprived of oxygen, they die. This is akin to the bone having suffered a stroke. The term *osteonecrosis* literally means "bone death." The term *avascular necrosis* is not as helpful. It is actually a redundancy because the word *necrosis* already implies death due to a lack of blood supply. Nevertheless, its abbreviation *AVN* is commonly used, probably because it is less of a mouthful than *osteonecrosis* or *avascular necrosis*. AVN, avascular necrosis, and osteonecrosis all denote the same condition.

For reasons that are not always completely understood, there are bones in the human body that are subject to seeing their blood supply interrupted. In the case of the thighbone (femur), it's not the whole bone that is at risk, just the two ends: the femoral head at the hip and the femoral condyles at the knee.

Sometimes there exists a clear-cut risk factor for a person to develop AVN: At particular risk are patients with sickle cell anemia and Gaucher's disease (a congenital "lipid storage" liver condition that allows large, vessel-clogging molecules to form), patients who have taken steroid medications (not including injections into tendons and joints), patients who ingest more than moderate amounts of alcohol, deep-sea divers who come up too quickly, and patients who have sustained specific types of trauma.

Some of these risk factors are relatively easy to understand: In sickle cell anemia the red cells clump together and clog small arteries called arterioles. If these arterioles represent the only source of blood for a particular section of bone, it's going to be a bad day for that piece of bone when those arterioles become clogged. The use of steroids is thought to increase the amount of tiny fat globules in the bloodstream, and these tiny globules can block an arteriole just like a clump of red cells.

It is important here to distinguish between different types of steroids. The steroids that can cause AVN are steroids taken by mouth or by injections into muscles (IM injections). Such steroids are given for a multitude of medical conditions including asthma, inflammatory arthritis (see above), organ transplants, head trauma, and chronic pain. Prednisone is typical of this category. Prednisone and related steroids are very different from the steroid preparations injected directly into a joint, such as Kenalog, Depo-Medrol, and Celestone. The latter are designed to work specifically on the joint that has been injected. They are not supposed to have so-called systemic effects, i.e., effects throughout the entire body. Sure, a small amount is certainly absorbed from the joint into the rest of the body, but by and large this small systemic dissemination has little effect. So with this second type of steroid you don't see the common side effects of prednisone such as swelling of the face, raising of blood sugar, and osteoporosis. Most significantly, you don't develop AVN from injections into a joint, assuming the injections are given at a reasonable frequency (for most patients three injections per year in a given joint would be considered reasonable).

Alcohol can affect the liver's ability to metabolize fats and it has been postulated that this can also lead to clogging of cer-

> **There exist many types of steroids. They do not all put you at risk for AVN.**

tain bone arterioles. Fractures can occasionally damage the arteries feeding a certain section of bone. This is particularly true of certain hip fractures. Divers who surface too quickly suffer from a condition called the bends. Nitrogen comes out of solution and forms bubbles. These bubbles, like clumped red cells and fat globules, can also clog arterioles.

But for half the patients suffering from AVN, there is no discernible cause. It just happens. When doctors cannot explain where a condition comes from, they term the condition *idiopathic*. If the doctor says you have idiopathic AVN, it means he or she can't identify any risk factor that would have caused your bone necrosis. Note that as more risk factors are identified, fewer people with AVN will be said to have the idiopathic variety. For example, I'm willing to bet that in the not too distant future we'll identify a certain gene that predisposes someone to the condition.

Investigators have noted that a bone with AVN builds up abnormal amounts of pressure. It remains to be determined whether this is the result or partly the cause of AVN.

How old are patients with AVN? Patients with AVN of the hip tend to be on the younger side, the average age being close to forty. Patients developing AVN of the knee are in their sixties or early seventies. Interestingly, though AVN can take months or years to develop, the pain often comes on *precipitously*, especially about the knee. Patients report pain coming out of the blue, a lightning bolt out of the sky. Hip AVN is much more common in men, but knee AVN is more common in women.

The natural progression of AVN. Sometimes the part of the bone that is affected by AVN is tiny. Bone being living tissue, it gobbles up the tiny dead part and replaces it with healthy, living bone. You may never have had a day of pain. If the part of the bone that is affected is bigger, you may develop pain, but the body may still be able to heal itself. Once it reaches a certain size, though, the condition progresses: Parts of the bone become rock hard, other parts become soft as the body tries to introduce new bone, and certain areas literally collapse (figure 1.2). The collapse usually takes place near the surface—in other words, near the articular cartilage. This is referred to as *subchondral collapse*. In the hip joint, the bone, instead of being convex, appears concave over the affected area (see also figure 7.1, page 96, to see what a normal femoral head looks like). This is called the *crescent sign*. Over time the cartilage deteriorates, and the bones on both sides of the joint rub together, producing a frankly arthritic picture.

The "staging" of AVN. AVN exists in varying degrees of severity. A number of staging classifications have developed over time to assist in communication and treatment. For example, your doctor might indicate in his report that you have Stage III AVN, thus communicating to any orthopedist the extent of your condition. There are four commonly accepted stages for AVN of the hip:

In Stage I, the AVN is not visible on the X-ray but is already visible on an MRI.

In Stage II, the dead bone is now apparent on the X-ray, being whiter than the surrounding bone.

In Stage III, the bone no longer has a smooth, round, convex shape. It has collapsed at the edge—the so-called crescent sign on a hip X-ray.

In Stage IV, the bones on either side of the joint have come together as the cartilage has deteriorated. To say that someone

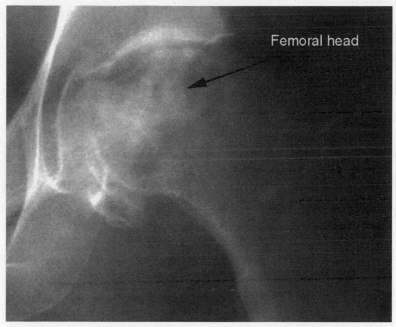

Figure 1.2 Osteonecrosis (avascular necrosis) of the hip. The normal femoral head is round. Note here how the bone has collapsed and the femoral head is no longer a smooth, round structure.

has Stage IV AVN is tantamount to saying that they now have arthritis.

Other classifications featuring groups and subgroups have been devised, but the stages I've outlined above are considered classic.

The treatment of AVN. Since we don't always know where AVN comes from, it isn't always easy to come up with a rational plan, and because there are multiple causes of AVN, it would make sense for the medical community to come up with a treatment specific to each cause. It hasn't happened yet.

Choices include using crutches to alleviate pain and to allow the bone to heal itself without collapsing, making holes in the bone (more on this shortly), bone grafting (bringing bone from elsewhere), applying electrical stimulation to the affected area, and replacing the joint.

The drilling of holes in the hip is called a *core decompression* since you take a core of bone out to decompress it. The concept of making holes in the bone comes from the observation that abnormal pressures build up in bones with AVN. This pressure causes pain and can contribute to cell death. Drilling holes in the affected area lowers the pressure. It may also stimulate the bone to remove the dead bone and replace it with healthy bone. At least so goes the theory. Since new bone is soft bone and soft bone is more prone to collapse, do you really want a large area of fresh, soft bone? Orthopedists have been debating this for years. There is no risk of aggravating the AVN by performing a core decompression, and so it is a commonly accepted procedure. But by making a hole in the shaft of the femur to gain access to the femoral head, the surgeon creates an area of weakness in the bone. This weakness predisposes you to a serious hip fracture should you take a misstep. Your surgeon will, therefore, have you walk with crutches for six to twelve weeks. Yes, back to the crutches. Cynics say that the core decompression is just a way of enforcing crutch walking that would otherwise be unacceptable to the patient.

Having made a hole in the bone, most surgeons are con-

> **The core decompression is designed to alleviate pressure within the bone. It is the modern equivalent of letting out the evil humors.**

tent to leave that hole unfilled. Another approach, though, is to fill the hole. Some surgeons have used a piece of fibula, the little bone that runs along the lower leg. But that piece of bone dies as soon as it is separated from its blood supply—that's what happens anytime you take a piece of bone out of someone. Other investigators have, therefore, harvested the fibula along with the main blood vessels feeding it. The vessels are then connected to arteries about the hip joint, thus maintaining the fibular graft alive. This is a relatively complex and time-consuming operation, but at least there is now a live piece of bone inside the femoral head. The extent to which this technique represents an improvement over the straightforward core decompression remains to be determined.

Electromagnetic stimulation was tried in the 1980s. The theory was that coursing a specific electromagnetic field across the affected hip would stimulate the healthy bone to replace the dead tissue. This was not as far-fetched as it seems, since electromagnetic stimulation has been shown to assist in the treatment of hard-to-heal fractures. Some investigators reported success early on, but this success has not been duplicated.

When all else fails and the AVN has reached Stage III or IV, a hip or knee replacement can be contemplated. The question that comes up in orthopedic circles is whether both sides of the hip joint need to be replaced. In other words, in addition to removing the afflicted femoral head, should the surgeon remove the articular cartilage covering the acetabulum (see chapters 7 and 8) and replace it with a cup? Here are the two sides of the argument: Only the femoral head is diseased, so why mess with the healthy cartilage on the acetabular side? Why not simply implant a partial hip replacement, a so-called *hemiarthroplasty*, the literal translation of which is "half" a replacement?

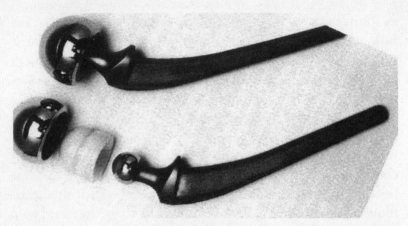

Figure 1.3 A partial hip replacement (*hemiarthroplasty*). The large, round metallic ball is the size of the femoral head that has been removed. This metallic ball is not fixed to the acetabulum (pelvis). Only the stem portion is fixed to bone. (*DePuy Orthopaedics, Inc.*)

In a hemiarthroplasty, the femoral head is replaced with a metallic ball that matches the size of the bone that was just removed (figure 1.3). This differs from a *total* hip replacement in two significant ways:

1. The acetabulum is left intact. No cup is implanted. The operation, therefore, takes less time than a *total* hip replacement.

2. The femoral head will usually measure somewhere between 44 and 54 millimeters as opposed to the 22-to-32-millimeter range found in a total hip replacement. The hip is, therefore, less likely to *dislocate* (pop out) after surgery (see chapters 8 and 18).

On the other hand, if a partial replacement is implanted, the large metallic ball will rub against the cartilage of the acetabulum. In a relatively young person, this type of repeated rubbing will eventually lead to the wearing out of the acetabular cartilage and to pain, pain that will require the surgeon to return into the hip to insert a cup. If this *conversion* from a partial to a total hip replacement takes place many, many years after the initial operation, the surgeon will have won his gamble, for the patient will have benefited from a pain-relieving procedure associated with a very low risk of dislocation. If the conversion needs to be done soon, however, it will be argued that the surgeon might as well have performed a total hip replacement right from the start! The problem, as you can see, is that no one knows in any given patient how long a partial replacement will last.

> **Surgery for hip fractures is one of the only life-saving orthopedic operations.**

So there you have it. You can see how the arguments balance out. I've tended to favor the total hip replacement approach, but have on occasion opted for the partial replacement in patients at particular risk for dislocations.

FEMORAL NECK FRACTURE

"People come into this world under the brim of the pelvis and leave it by the neck of the femur."

This is a medical adage that goes back many centuries, as hip fractures were terminal events until the advent of surgery. An older person immobilized by the pain of a hip fracture would develop bedsores, pneumonia, or urinary infections, and die. Thus, the primary goal of hip fracture surgery is to save the person's life. The second goal is to allow the patient to walk again. The third goal is to restore the patient to her prior level of function. Sometimes a family will be disappointed that Grandma isn't good as new. But if she's alive, let alone walking, she's already benefited from one of the miracles of modern medicine.

When a person sustains a hip fracture, you can quibble about whether she fell and broke her hip or vice versa. The most current thinking is that most of the time the impact against the ground causes the fracture. In fact, padded girdles exist that may minimize the risk of such a fracture, but they are neither widely available nor prescribed. There are issues of cost (who will pay for such a device?), acceptance (no one likes to think of themselves as being so old and frail that they need to wear padded protection around both hips), and effectiveness (no study has demonstrated the exact extent to which these pads prevent fractures). From an orthopedic point of view, whether the fall or the fracture comes first is irrelevant—the result is the same.

A hip fracture is a fracture of the upper portion of the femur (see chapter 7). American orthopedic surgeons (aka orthopedists) treat 250,000 of these per year, and the numbers will increase as Baby Boomers discover about ten years from now that marijuana expands the mind but not the bone.

A hip can break in one of three places: the femoral neck, the intertrochanteric area, or the subtrochanteric region (figure 1.4). Each type of fracture presents the surgeon with a different set of challenges. The intertrochanteric and the subtrochanteric fractures are fixed with plates, screws, or rods, the

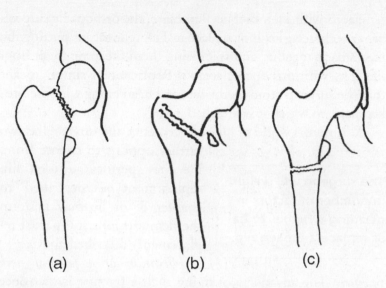

Figure 1.4 Hip fractures. (a) The normal hip looks somewhat like a scoop of ice cream on a cone. In a femoral neck fracture a crack appears between the ice cream and the cone, and, in more severe cases, the ice cream appears to have completely fallen off the cone. (b) The intertrochanteric fracture. (c) The subtrochanteric fracture.

so-called *open reduction and internal fixation*, abbreviated *ORIF*. These procedures range from simple to maddeningly complex. The femoral neck fractures are a breed apart. The femoral neck is a narrow structure with relatively little soft, *cancellous*, healing type of bone. Therefore, it is at risk for a nonunion, a fracture that refuses to heal. Fractures of the femoral neck are also associated with the potential disruption of the blood vessels supplying the femoral head. Fractures of the femoral neck are, therefore, associated with a condition called *osteonecrosis*, whereby a section of bone loses its blood supply and dies (see the previous section).

Faced with a femoral neck fracture, the orthopedic surgeon has two choices: Fix it or replace it. Fixing it means putting the pieces back together and stabilizing them (keeping them from moving) with orthopedic screws. Replacement simply means that the surgeon removes the femoral head along with the broken neck to which it is attached.

Within the world of hip replacements, the surgeon has two further options to choose from. He may perform a total hip replacement as described in chapter 8, or he may perform the hemiarthroplasty (partial replacement) described above.

> **The surgeon will weigh a number of factors in deciding whether to fix or replace a broken hip.**

Fixation of a femoral neck fracture. The advantage of fixing such a fracture is that once the fracture has healed—and assuming that no osteonecrosis develops—you are good as new. It's as if the fracture never occurred. Of course, there are exceptions. Older patients are frequently knocked down a peg even with perfect healing of their fracture. If they were excellent walkers prior to the injury and surgery, they are now good walkers. Good walkers become fair walkers, etc. But younger patients are often close to being good as new. Once the fracture has healed, there are no restrictions on activities. True, the screws or plate may need to be removed one day (mostly in younger patients), and this will require a period of crutch walking, but those restrictions are temporary. The three downsides to fixing a femoral neck fracture are that (1) you may need to use crutches for six to twelve weeks, (2) the bone may not heal, and (3) the femoral head may go on to osteonecrosis. The last two scenarios require a trip back to the operating room for a hip replacement.

Hip replacement. With hip replacement surgery, you don't have to worry about the bone not healing (there are no longer two pieces of bone that need to heal together!) and osteonecrosis is not a concern because the part of the bone that dies (the femoral head) has been removed! And in an older patient, even crutch walking is not an issue because the surgeon will use a technique that doesn't require it.

However, hip replacements have their own set of complications. They can become infected, they can dislocate, and over time, they can loosen and wear out.

Choosing the right operation. First, the surgeon has to decide whether to fix or replace your hip. The factors he will consider include your age, your level of activity, and the "displacement" of the fracture. The older you are, the more likely he is to pick a joint replacement. This is because the older patient is going to be less tolerant of hobbling for two to three months only to find that she needs to return to the operating room. A hip replacement in an older patient is also less likely to loosen or wear out in his or her lifetime.

The surgeon will also lean toward a hip replacement if you are on the less active side, for the less active you are, the less likely your hip is to loosen or wear out.

The specific nature of the fracture is also a factor. The fracture can be of the *nondisplaced* type, whereby the fracture consists of a simple crack akin to a crack in the wall (figure 1.4). The two pieces are still connected and haven't moved relative to each other. The femoral head can be *impacted*, i.e., pushed into the femoral neck as a scoop of ice cream might be pushed into a cone. Finally, the fracture can be *displaced:* The bone has snapped like a pencil, and the two fragments might as well be in different rooms. In the case of the nondisplaced and of the impacted fracture, the surgeon is dealing with a relatively stable situation. With a little luck, the fracture could heal without any surgical intervention. The surgeon need only place a few orthopedic pins across the fracture to prevent displacement of the fracture, something that might happen if you fell again or took a misstep. Clearly, in the setting of the nondisplaced and of the impacted fracture, a hip replacement is overkill. The more difficult decision comes with the displaced fracture, and this is where the surgeon will review your age and your level of activity. The older and less active you are, the more likely he is to recommend a replacement; the younger and more active you are, the more likely he is to recommend fixation.

If he's decided to replace your hip, your surgeon must now decide between a total hip replacement and a hemiarthroplasty (see figure 1.3). In the United States, he will choose a hemiarthroplasty 99 percent of the time. This is because most patients who break their hip are elderly.

A hemiarthroplasty is a quicker operation than a total hip replacement and therefore theoretically safer (less anesthesia time, less bleeding, less exposure to the air).

The issue of the metal ball rubbing against the acetabular cartilage is less likely to be a significant factor in an older, lighter, less active patient.

A hemiarthroplasty is less likely to dislocate (pop out) than a total hip replacement. This is because the femoral head is larger in a hemiarthroplasty, and larger heads are less prone to dislocate (see chapters 8 and 18).

But an argument can be made for performing a total hip replacement. Some patients who fracture their hip may also have some early arthritis. If they are still relatively young and active (a healthy seventy-year-old woman actuarially speaking, still has many years to live!), the hemiarthroplasty may become painful in short order. The hemiarthroplasty will need to be changed to a total hip replacement. This is called a *conversion* even though there is no religion involved. Converting a hemiarthroplasty to a total hip replacement is much harder than performing a total hip replacement right off the bat. It is associated with many of the risks of revision hip replacement discussed in chapter 9.

In a patient with underlying arthritis, the situation is really a no-brainer, and in this particular situation (fracture plus arthritis) the surgeon will, in fact, get reimbursed more for a total hip replacement than for a hemiarthroplasty (this is because "arthritis" codes pay more than fracture codes). The difficult decision-making comes in the setting of a pure fracture devoid of any arthritic component in a patient who is reasonably active in the community. In theory, the surgeon has to weigh all of the above factors and has to discuss them with you before coming to a decision. In practice, a diagnosis of a displaced femoral neck fracture will nearly automatically lead to a hemiarthroplasty. The urgent circumstances of the fracture and admission to the hospital don't allow for much discussion.

> **"The sun doesn't set on a hip fracture."**

This is another time-honored adage, going back to the earliest days of hip surgery. Since prolonged bed rest leads to medical complications, it was recognized early on that prompt surgical treatment and early mobilization of the patient out of bed into a chair saves lives. Ideally, the subject should have her fracture surgically addressed on the same day as her admission to the hospital.

In the real world, the surgery often takes place the following day or evening. If the patient is not "medically cleared," i.e., suffers from a condition that won't allow surgery, the surgery is delayed until that condition is cleared up or stabilized. But generally speaking, complications increase with the length of the delay.

Here then is the dilemma: Operate soon and avoid bedsores, pneumonia, and urinary tract infections, or operate later to evaluate and fully understand, say, the temperature that your mother has been running, or her cardiac function. Your family doctor and the anesthesiologist will usually vote for the latter. This is in part because they don't want intraoperative complications (who does?) and in part because they don't always appreciate the risks associated with delaying the surgery.

> **Can you *believe* they missed my mother's fracture?**

HOW DOCTORS MISS FEMORAL NECK FRACTURES

"Can you believe they missed my mother's fracture over at City General? Sent her right out of the emergency room!!! We took her to County General a few days later, where they said the fracture was very clear."

If I had a dollar for each time I've heard this story . . .
So how does this happen?
First of all, missed fractures occur in every part of the body. And the reason is simple: They don't necessarily show up initially. They start off as a tiny, invisible crack. The body's initial

response to a fracture is to "resorb" bone at the edges of the fracture; i.e., bone at the edge of the fracture is taken away. Remember: Bone is a living tissue that is constantly breaking itself down and rebuilding. This resorption of bone at the fracture edges leads the fracture to temporarily widen, thus making it more visible. Consequently, a fracture is sometimes more visible on Day 4 than it is on the day of the injury.

For many parts of the body, missing a little fracture is of no great importance. If the doctor treats you for a bad bruise of the shoulder or a bad sprain of the ankle, the treatment will be the same as for a small, hard-to-see fracture. But the hip is different—at least the femoral neck portion of the hip. A small crack across the femoral neck can be treated with pins that look like knitting needles. These are put in through a small skin incision, the blood loss is negligible, you can put all your weight on the leg immediately, and healing is essentially guaranteed.

> **Not everyone is equally satisfied with their hip replacement . . .**

teed. If you are young and healthy enough, it can be an outpatient procedure. If the crack goes unrecognized, however, the neck of the hip can snap in two. Now you need a hip replacement—a very different operation. It is, therefore, critical for emergency room doctors to detect the slightest fracture of the femoral neck. The way for them to do so in the twenty-first century is to obtain an MRI. The MRI is the most sensitive test for a hip fracture; in other words, it is the test most likely to detect a fracture. Although I've gone on record as stating that MRIs are seriously abused in the United States (see *What Your Doctor May* Not *Tell You About Knee Pain and Surgery*, Warner, 2002), the finding of a normal X-ray in the face of severe hip pain readily justifies an MRI. Orthopedists as well as a growing number of emergency room doctors will, therefore, quickly resort to an MRI in this setting. If you are not able to undergo an MRI, a CT scan is the next best option.

PATIENT SATISFACTION IS IN THE EYE OF THE BEHOLDER

Who is more satisfied with her hip replacement? The patient suffering from arthritis or the one who's broken her hip?

The one with arthritis.

The patient with arthritis has been suffering a long time. Pain walking. Pain going up and down stairs. Pain clipping toenails and putting on socks. Any significant relief is welcome. If the pain score goes down from a 10 to a 3, the patient thanks his lucky stars. If the operated leg is a little long (see chapters 8 and 18), so be it.

Not so the patient with a hip fracture. The day before sustaining her fracture, Mrs. Smith had no pain whatsoever in her hip. Her leg lengths were identical. She expects the surgeon to return her to that exact state, especially if she is relatively young. A pain score of 3 is not as acceptable nor is a slight difference in her leg lengths. Also, in the setting of a fracture the surgeon hasn't had the time to review these subtleties with his new patient (nor has the patient had the time to read this book!).

Summary: Arthritis is the number one condition necessitating a *total* hip replacement. Partial hip replacements are most commonly used for hip fractures. AVN is relatively uncommon compared to arthritis and hip fractures. Both total and partial hip replacements are utilized for this condition.

Chapter 2

❧❧

Nonoperative Alternatives

Presumably you've passed the point of trying more nonoperative treatment. In the companion book, *What Your Doctor May Not Tell You About Knee Pain And Surgery* (Warner, 2002), I reviewed some of the hanky-panky that goes on in the world of knee pain, especially as it pertains to bogus reports of "torn cartilage" and the resulting unnecessary surgery. But few people undergo unwarranted joint replacement surgery. If your doctor tells you that you need a joint replacement, chances are good that he is correct. The question here is one of timing. Arthritis pain typically comes and goes. The patient visiting the doctor with an arthritic flare-up will agree to just about anything, and occasionally an unscrupulous surgeon will take advantage of that by proposing surgery. You, therefore, want to make sure that you've had repeated and prolonged

> **If you suffer from arthritis or osteonecrosis, it's not a question of whether you need a joint replacement but *when* you'll need one.**

flare-ups before you agree to joint replacement surgery and will want to have tried a number of the options listed below.

Caveat emptor: Remedies that allegedly require three months of continued use before they can be effective may be taking advantage of the fact that, in that period of time, most arthritic flare-ups will have quieted down on their own.[1]

Rest. This may seem obvious, but people sometimes want to "work through" the pain. An arthritic flare-up demands rest. Gentle exercises can be resumed once the acute pain has abated.

Heat and cold treatment. Although they are opposites, both heat and cold can be soothing. People generally like to be given specific formulas (for example, "Do this for ten minutes, then do that for fifteen minutes"), but when it comes to heat and cold, there is no right or wrong. It's a question of what works best for each individual person. I generally recommend ten minutes of one followed by ten minutes of the other. "Should the heat be moist or dry?" is a frequently asked question. Personally, I have not noted a difference, although individual patients have indicated a preference for one or the other. Some people, for example, feel particularly well in a warm bath. Beware of overdoing it! I've seen people *burn* themselves with a heating pad. Taking a sedative, imbibing an alcoholic beverage, and falling asleep with an electric heating pad around your knee is not a good idea. When it comes to cold, the key is not to place ice directly on the skin. Believe it or not, you can get *frostbite*! Place a towel or wrap an elastic bandage between the ice and your skin. There are some com-

---

1. This chapter has been adapted from *What Your Doctor May Not Tell You About Knee Pain and Surgery* (Warner, 2002).

mercially available neoprene wraps that can house a gel pack. This pack can be cooled or heated. In fact, two gel packs can be used, so that while one is being used, the other can be either cooled or heated.

MEDICATIONS

Oral Medications (Pills)

These fall into many categories:

Analgesics. These simply mask the pain. There is nothing wrong with that, as long as you don't go out and abuse your arthritic joint while you're feeling better. These include acetaminophen (brand name, Tylenol) and tramadol (Ultram). Acetaminophen is an over-the-counter medication and is *relatively* safe. Nevertheless, it can have side serious effects that you don't even feel (e.g., liver damage), and you should inform your doctor if you find yourself taking this medication on a regular basis (I feel that this is true for any medication or nutritional supplement).

Anti-inflammatories. Nonsteroidal anti-inflammatory drugs (NSAIDs) calm pain by chemically quieting the irritation associated with arthritis. Aspirin is the granddaddy of all NSAIDs. In ancient Greece women in labor were advised to chew on the leaves of the willow tree, as the salicin in the leaves would alleviate their pain. A salicin derivative has become the aspirin we know today. It is common wisdom that, had it been discovered just in the last few decades, it would never have been approved as an over-the-counter drug. It has multiple effects, it can interact with other medications, and it can adversely affect important biological functions for many weeks.

For example, aspirin compromises platelets that help the blood to clot. This is very useful when aspirin is used as a blood thinner, but it is a major problem when blood thinning is contraindicated. You should definitely let your doctor know that you are taking aspirin when he or she prescribes *any other* medication.

Since the introduction of aspirin, dozens of NSAIDs have appeared on and disappeared from the market. Each one naturally claims to be more powerful and have fewer side effects than the existing ones. These side effects include stomach ulcers, which can hurt and cause serious bleeding, and more insidious damage to various organ systems such as the kidneys. The possibility has even been raised that NSAIDs can harm articular cartilage—the very root of the arthritis problem. I have not personally noted clinical evidence of this, but it is a point worth keeping in mind. The newest class of NSAIDs is the so-called COX-2 inhibitor (valdecoxib [brand name, Bextra], celecoxib [Celebrex], refecoxib [Vioxx], and, in standard doses, meloxican [Mobic]), which are even less likely to cause ulcers than the recent NSAIDs already being touted as mild on the stomach. Note that the COX-2 NSAIDs are not better pain relievers than the other NSAIDs. So if your current NSAID works and you are not at risk for ulcers (speak to your doctor about this), I would not switch. Not to mention that Bextra, Celebrex, and Vioxx are quite expensive.

The following is another common misconception: NSAIDs will reduce swelling. If the knee is swollen due to the irritation of arthritis, then yes, maybe. But if the swelling is the result of an injury, no! You might take ibuprofen, for instance, for the pain of a sprained ankle, but don't expect it to control that goose egg on the outside of your foot! NSAIDs control the pain of irritation but *do not remove any water* that has accumulated. The swelling from an injury will resolve only with rest, elevation, cold, compression, tincture of time, powder of patience, and extract of expectation.

Keep in mind that patents run out after a few years. If you wonder why you don't hear of a great medication after a while, it's either because serious side effects have been discovered and the drug has been pulled off the market, or more likely, the patent has run out, and advertising is no longer cost-effective. One medication that I have found to be effective in treating arthritic pain is naproxen. It is convenient (twice-a-day dosage) and has been around a very long time. In its generic form it is relatively inexpensive and you are not likely to wake up to the news that it has been pulled from the market. Remarkably, certain HMOs and insurance companies will not cover naproxen. They will, however, cover brand-only, expensive NSAIDs. Go figure.

Having said this, in patients over the age of fifty-five, I will probably start with either a low dose of naproxen or an NSAID that is milder on the stomach.

One point that is remarkably unappreciated is that you can combine an NSAID with an analgesic. For example, you can take naproxen with breakfast and dinner and, in between, add

> **Newer medications tend to be expensive. Your surgeon may not be attuned to this, and if cost is important to you, speak up.**

acetaminophen to manage more isolated flare-ups (check with your doctor for the exact dosage).

Should you be asking for the very latest NSAID? Not necessarily. Every new car model is better than the last one, but the same doesn't apply to medications or medical devices. True, our government demands stringent tests, but there are still surprises. Remember Duract? Of course not. It came out briefly in the late 1990s, and was gone before you could say "complication." People got touchy about a few deaths here and there, and in the twitch of a liver enzyme, it was gone. Mind you, there may have been a little overreaction on the part of public. It really wasn't clear that the deaths were related to the medication, but the point remains that there can be surprises with new medications.

Newer medications tend to be expensive. Your surgeon may not be attuned to this, and if cost is important to you, speak up.

Then there are the new medications that aren't new at all. Take the case of the pain reliever Vicoprofen. Vicoprofen consists of two separate generic medications put together: hydrocodone and ibuprofen. Hydrocodone is a strong, time-honored narcotic, and ibuprofen is a classic NSAID available as Motrin, Advil, Nuprin, or simply ibuprofen. These two medications are relatively cheap as generics. Although hydrocodone and ibuprofen are inexpensive on their own, one enterprising manufacturer has combined the two medications to create the more expensive Vicoprofen! You'd have thought, "Nah, that'll never work." Who would pay a lot of money for a pill that consists of two inexpensive medications? Well, wrong again. This has been a popular medication. I suppose that for some people the convenience of swallowing one larger pill rather than two smaller pills is worth the extra expense. You be the judge.

And by the way, Vicoprofen isn't alone. Many prescriptions and over-the-counter medications are pricey combinations of inexpensive products. Read the label and check with your pharmacist.

Steroids. Steroids are a large class of medications derived from hormones produced by the human adrenal glands (one adrenal gland rests over each kidney). The word *steroid* is actually an abbreviation of *corticosteroid, cortico-* referring to the cortex, i.e., outer layer, of the adrenal gland. It is important to note that steroids used for the pain of arthritis are different from anabolic steroids taken by some athletes. Cortisone was one of the original steroids, and the word *cortisone* is still used colloquially to denote any type of steroid. Steroids are strong anti-inflammatory medications that work by suppressing the formation of pain-producing compounds such as prostaglandins. However, they are associated with a long list of potential side effects. These include stomach ulcers, fluid retention, the raising of blood sugar, osteonecrosis (see chapter 1), and osteoporosis, to name but a few. Not everyone suffers from these side effects. The likelihood of developing one or more side effects depends on the dose of the medication and on the length of time the medication is taken. Despite their potential side effects, steroids are sometimes the only medications that will be effective, and doctors do still prescribe them. Interestingly, though the word *cortisone* is commonly used, I don't believe that it is still in clinical practice—at least not in the United States. Indeed, despite the fact that cortisone conjures up nasty

> A number of narcotics are packaged with acetaminophen (Tylenol), often labeled as APAP. Therefore, do not take acetaminophen on top of your prescribed pain medication without checking with your doctor.

things in people's minds, it is actually relatively weak. Prednisone, on the other hand, is much stronger and is a commonly prescribed steroid.

Narcotics. An arthritic flare-up can be excruciating, and on a short-term basis, it is reasonable to take a narcotic. A narcotic, or opioid, is a compound closely related in chemical structure to opium, or its derivative, morphine. Most narcotics are derived from natural extracts, but a few, like demerol and fentanyl, are synthetic. Endorphins are narcotics that are manufactured by our own bodies. Characteristically, this class of medication provides good pain relief, sleepiness, a feeling of well-being, and constipation.

In the long run, it is not advisable to use narcotics, for the reasons most of us know: They are addictive and they become less effective with time. One is said to become *tolerant* to them. If you take narcotics, keep in mind that they can be constipating and can make you drowsy. The most common narcotics are combined with acetaminophen or aspirin. Check the label. If the abbreviation *APAP* appears, you will know that your medication includes acetaminophen, in which case it is not a good idea to take even more acetaminophen. The same goes for aspirin, which might be labeled *ASA.*

Not all narcotics are of equal strength. Tylenol 3, which contains codeine, lies at the lower end of the spectrum and in the street is referred to as T3. This narcotic often suffices for patients suffering from their first bouts of arthritis. Tylenol 4 contains the same amount of Tylenol (acetaminophen), but twice the amount of codeine. Vicodin is a combination of hydrocodone and acetaminophen. Vicodin ES contains the same amount of acetaminophen but more hydrocodone. Percocet is similar to Vicodin, except that the hydrocodone has been replaced by another narcotic of essentially equal strength—oxycodone. In Percodan the oxycodone is joined to aspirin rather than acetaminophen. Because of their greater recognition and street value when compared to Vicodin, the doctor needs to fill out a special prescription for Percocet and Percodan.

Note: Hydrocodone and oxycodone contain no codeine, though the words sound similar (Lennon and Lenin were very different people).

The next step up from Vicodin and Percocet is Dilaudid. This is usually reserved for the patient with chronic pain who has become *tolerant* to lesser narcotics. In my practice, a patient in need of Dilaudid gets a consultation from a pain specialist, usually an anesthesiologist with knowledge and interest in patients with chronic pain.

Having said all of this, all narcotics from mildest to strongest are prescription medications. You cannot obtain them over-the-counter.

Consider this little-known fact: Pain medications work best when the pain *just* starts coming on. Sometimes, it doesn't pay to be a hero. When you feel the pain coming on, take something for it.

Injections

As unappealing as they are to most people, injections into the knee still have a place. These usually consist of a combination of a numbing agent (e.g., Novocain) and a steroid, a class of compounds that suppress swelling and irritation. You'll be interested to know that not all steroids are equivalent. Some are more expensive than others, and in my opinion, this is an example of getting what you pay for: The more expensive ones are stronger, last longer, and don't leave a dandruff-like residue in the knee. I use Celestone (betamethasone) when it is available. (It has not uncommonly been on back-order, in other words, unavailable.)

There are downsides to steroid injections: Not only are they not curative, but they make the tissues less healthy and more prone to infection. There is, therefore, a limit to how many injections one can prescribe. I limit knee joint injections to three per year. Note that injections affect the site that has been injected, and have limited impact on other sites. If you've had three shoulder injections, you can still receive a knee injection. The steroid quiets the inflammation. It does so for a variable period of time, which is why some people think of such injections as miracles while others grumble that they are a waste of time. Note that steroid injections in standard doses have *not* been associated with osteonecrosis.

Injections into the hip are also possible, but slightly more involved. Except in the thinnest of people, the hip joint is deep below the skin and more readily missed by the needle. A longer needle is required, and ideally the injection should be performed under fluoroscopy (a continuous X-ray), to ensure that the tip of the needle is where it is supposed to be. I will not uncommonly send patients to the radiology department of the hospital for hip injections.

There exist a class of injections unrelated to steroids that were introduced in 1998. These injections consist of a gooey, synthetic version of the hyaluronic acid that your own joints make. Injecting these products into the knee is akin to adding oil to a machine (for now these injections are approved only for the knee). The patient needs to come for a series of three weekly shots. The manufacturers have found that cartilage growth can be stimulated by these injections. It is not clear to what extent this is a clinically significant finding, in other words, to what extent people will benefit from this feature. In my experience, these injections work best in patients whose arthritis is not terribly ad-vanced, but I have seen excep-tions in both directions. When the injections work, they remain effective for three months to a year. The injec-tions are pricey, and not all in-surances cover them.[2]

> **If the tip of the needle is in the fat pad, the injection will be painful. Therefore, if the injection is quite painful, the needle may be in wrong place.**

You should be aware of the following technical point: There exists a structure in your knee called the fat pad. It varies in size from person to person.

If the tip of the needle is in the fat pad, the injection will be painful and the hyaluronic acid will never make it into its target, namely the cavity we call the joint. The injection should be performed by someone with experience in this area.

NUTRITIONAL SUPPLEMENTS

It would be very appealing to prescribe an oral medication that leads to the regeneration of worn-out cartilage. The manufac-turers of two products—glucosamine and chondroitin sulfate—have made such a claim, and there is a school of thought that the

2. Some insurance companies have been known to be devious. They claim to cover the prod-ucts, but only on condition that the patient not be a candidate for a joint replacement. Yet every patient with knee or hip arthritis is a candidate for a joint replacement! If the potential need for a replacement is in any way stated in the patient's record, coverage is denied!

two products should be taken together. Even the most fervent proponents recognize that the pain relief does not start until the products have been used regularly for at least one month (some say three months). Since both products exist in the body, though not necessarily in that exact form, they cannot be called drugs. They are classified as nutritional supplements. The good news is that they are not under the control of the FDA, and scientific validation is not required. They can be promoted and sold without having to wait the many years it takes for the FDA to determine that something is safe and effective. The bad news is that is that they are not under the control of the FDA, and scientific validation is not required. They can be promoted and sold without having to wait the many years it takes for the FDA to determine that something is safe and effective! If the products are found to be ineffective, many people will have wasted an awful lot of money. Fortunately, so far it appears that the products are safe, and a smattering of scientific articles suggesting that these supplements are indeed effective in calming pain are beginning to appear. Major side effects to these compounds have not been widely reported. Anecdotally, a number of my patients swear by these products. Therefore, if money is not an issue (the supplements can be expensive), I don't discourage my patients from trying them. But one has to keep in mind the fact that arthritic flare-ups quiet down on their own (see above), and so pain relief may have nothing to do with a supplement's efficacy. Also there can be placebo effects.

A *placebo* is a treatment that the doctor recognizes as having no medicinal value. Yet, if the patient believes enough in the treatment (*placebo* comes from the Latin "I shall please"), this may be enough to ensure success. It's a case of "mind over matter." Although I am discussing this in the context of nutritional supplements where there has been little scientific validation, the placebo effect can be manifest with *any* treatment, even surgery!

DIET

Rattlesnake meat, vinegar, honey, and white meat have all been touted as arthritis remedies, whereas tomatoes, eggplant, potatoes, sweets, and dairy products get the thumbs-down. That is, if you believe in all this. I don't. It would be all too easy if a little rattlesnake and honey sandwich did the trick. Don't get me wrong: Many of our scientific remedies come from natural products. If aspirin can come from the willow tree, then perhaps there is something medicinal about honey. But if this were the case, it would no longer be a secret, and right now if honey or vinegar is effective against arthritis, it's certainly a secret to me.

PHYSICAL THERAPY (PT)

Physical therapy is a broad field including exercises and modalities designed to promote motion and decrease pain. The exercises themselves can be divided into the stretching and the strengthening types. When physical therapy is suggested to patients with arthritis, they occasionally have the mistaken impression that they are being sent for a strengthening program, complete with pushing, pulling, huffing, and puffing. This is not appealing. However, PT in the setting of knee and hip arthritis is more of the *stretching and modality* variety (see "Arthritis and Exercise," below), though *painless* strengthening is a welcome addition.

An arthritic joint tends to get stiff. This is the body's natural response to arthritis. *Moving* an arthritic joint is what hurts.

If the knee could be rendered completely stiff to the point where it didn't move at all, there would be no pain. There are problems with the body's attempt to freeze the joint: (1) The joint is never completely stiff, and so the pain persists. (2) A stiff joint doesn't work very well. (3) The stiffness is, to some extent, imparted by the chronic tensing of muscles, and this itself can contribute to the person's pain. A portion of PT, therefore, involves restoring reasonable motion to the knee or hip.

In addition to applying heat and cold, which patients can do on their own at home, PT can involve modalities such as ultrasound and, in more sophisticated settings, ionto- or phonophoresis. This is a process where drugs are applied to the skin and electrochemically led to diffuse through the skin. In my experience, these modalities tend to work better on problems that are relatively superficial (e.g., tendinitis) than on arthritis, which lives down deep inside the joint. Nevertheless, the process can be worth trying.

> **Yes, people with arthritis should exercise!**

Massage. The tendons and muscles about an arthritic joint tend to be stiff and sore. Massage aids in the stretching of these structures and thereby soothes the hip or knee. It also soothes the soul. This is not an insignificant factor in the overall treatment of the patient whose pain has rendered him or her tense and irritable.

Arthritis and Exercise

Patients with knee arthritis tend not to exercise. Exercise hurts. There is also the fear that exercise will aggravate the arthritis. Nevertheless, not only is exercise allowed in this setting, but it is to be encouraged—not just for the sake of the hip or knee but for the additional cardiovascular benefits of aerobic exercise.

We are not talking about just any exercise. Jumping, twisting, and high-impact activities will tend to increase the pain. At the other extreme, water exercises are wonderful. The body is buoyant, and therefore, by definition, less weight is placed across the hip and knee. Running, which on land could be painful, may suddenly be quite tolerable in a pool. It can be carried out in the shallow end of a pool or, with special flotation belts, in the deep end. Likewise, kicking and jumping exercises are more readily prescribed in water. These strengthen the muscles (this makes the knee feel more secure), stretch the structures about the knee, contribute to cardiovascular fitness, and provide a sense of well-being. The water temperature should be comfortable, if not initially, at least within a few moments of exercising. If the water is too cold, the muscles will become even tenser and more painful.

For land exercises, cushioned shoes should be worn. Use of a treadmill is reasonable since the surface is relatively soft. The use of an exercise bicycle is by and large a neutral exercise: It won't help, and it won't hurt. Running is controversial. At one point, it was felt to cause arthritis, but recent studies suggest that in a perfectly normal knee, running does not promote arthritis. In a knee that is already arthritic, it may be a different story. I would tend to discourage running for someone who is quite bowlegged or knock-kneed.

SHOE WEAR

In a painfully arthritic hip or knee, every jarring step hurts. Classic, leather-soled shoes with hard rubber heels don't help the situation. Wearing shoes with softer heels, such as running shoes, or inserting a cushioned insole can help. If you use an insole, make sure it is thick enough. Some foam insoles collapse like tissue paper and provide minimal cushioning. Silicone (not silicon) inserts are more durable and provide more cushioning.

CANES, STICKS, AND THE LIKE

Getting a patient to use a cane is a measure of how good a salesman the doctor is. Other than "orthopedic" shoes, no other treatment option has such a stigma attached to it. Where knee replacement surgery is high-tech, a cane just makes you look old—or so people feel. Naturally, men take to canes better than women. There are some very elegant canes, and men with canes can still conjure up a certain aura. A hiking stick may be more acceptable, though not necessarily when shopping down Fifth Avenue. Other alternatives include a golf umbrella or a shopping cart. No matter how you disguise it, though, a cane is a hard sell. And yet, there is no question that using some kind of support will take pressure off the knee and provide some pain relief. A cane also addresses the *unsteadiness* some people feel as a result of their pain. If you've finally given in to using a cane, at least use it correctly!

How to Use a Cane

If you resort to a cane, walking stick, or hiking stick, you need to know three things:

1. If you are using the cane for *hip* pain, place the cane in the hand *opposite* the side of your painful hip. If

your right hip hurts, hold the cane with the left hand. For knee pain, it doesn't matter as much.

2. The cane moves forward at the same time as the painful leg. Let us continue with the example of right hip pain. As you move forward and your right heel strikes the ground, you should be leaning to the left onto your cane. It takes a little practice, but no harder than rubbing the top of your head and your belly at the same time.

3. The top of the cane should be no higher than the bottom of your pants pocket. Most of the canes I see are too long. Your elbow should have just a little bend in it, so that you can really lean on it.

BRACES

Arthritis pain is partly the result of two bones rubbing. A snug knee support or tightly wrapped elastic bandage can minimize such rubbing, and assuage pain. That is the theory. In my experience, braces and wraps have a low probability of success. With the use of tight wraps, there is the added concern that the blood circulation might be compromised, though this would be of concern only in patients suffering from vascular disease. Because these supports are inexpensive, they can be worth trying. They are available in surgical supply stores (where you purchase items such as crutches and back braces) and in large drugstores. They come in various colors and materials. A common material is neoprene, the same neoprene that scuba diving wet suits are made of—and with the same result: The knee feels warm. This is desirable in the dead of a cold winter but barely tolerable in the heat of summer. Other supports are merely elastic and provide less warmth. They can, however, be as snug as neoprene. Some supports come with straps that allow you to fine-tune the tightness of your support. If a strapless support feels just right, you don't need the straps. If a given support tends to slide down your leg and the smaller size is too tight, consider the larger size that comes with straps and use the straps to firm things up.

For patients whose arthritis is relatively mild and confined to just the inner aspect of the knee (medial arthritis), there exist bulky, long leg braces that imperceptibly push the knee into a less bowlegged and more knock-kneed position, thus taking pressure and pain off the inner aspect of the knee. In this specific situation, a brace can be safe and effective, especially if applied to a relatively thin, muscular leg.

ACUPUNCTURE

The philosophy of acupuncture is based on the premise that human life flows along fourteen major meridians (channels). Each meridian governs a major organ system. Blockage of a meridian leads to pain or dysfunction while selective stimulation of meridians restores equilibrium and health. Acupuncture is an accepted adjunct to anesthesia, and I have occasionally seen patients obtain satisfactory relief from acupuncture in the setting of an arthritic joint. As with every other option listed, it is not a cure.

Chapter 3

Operative Alternatives to Joint Replacement Surgery

THE HIP

If a total hip replacement has been suggested, you probably suffer from arthritis, avascular necrosis, or a hip fracture, conditions that are described in chapter 1.

The major surgical alternative to a total hip replacement is an *osteotomy,* a procedure that cuts the bone and changes its direction. The concept is simple: The femoral head of the hip joint is round like a lightbulb (see chapter 1). If only part of the femoral head is worn out, the surgeon can turn it so that a healthy part now articulates with the pelvis. This was popu-

> **A hip osteotomy changes the direction of the hipbone in order to take stress off the damaged part of the joint.**

lar in the days before hip replacement surgery, and there exist many treatises describing the techniques, indications, and complications of such an approach. A variation on this is the *pelvic osteotomy*. Instead of cutting the femur (thighbone), the surgeon cuts the pelvis to reshape or redirect it.

The main advantages of an osteotomy are that once it has healed, and assuming that significant pain relief has been obtained, there are no limitations on the patient's activities and there is no risk of a dislocation, one of the major risks of hip replacement surgery (see chapters 17 and 18). Moreover, an "osteotomized" hip can remain pain-free for ten or more years.

Osteotomies of the hip are infrequently recommended in the United States for four reasons: First, they are technically demanding and are best performed by surgeons who perform them frequently. However, few American surgeons perform them frequently and few surgeons are likely to recommend a procedure that they are not comfortable with. Second, the recovery can be lengthy since the cut bone must heal. Third, osteotomies are hardly a guarantee of a pain-free hip. Finally, the anatomic distortion created by the osteotomy may make the eventual hip replacement more complex and more prone to failure. The surgeon may, therefore, elect to get twenty years out of a hip replacement and cross the next bridge when he gets to it.

> **A fusion melds two bones together. Motion disappears and so does pain. The lack of motion, however, can make certain mundane activities cumbersome.**

Because a hip replacement placed into a young patient is likely to wear out in the subject's lifetime, and because redo hip replacement surgery is riskier than the original operation, an osteotomy remains a serious consideration for the rare patients suffering from arthritis in their twenties or thirties.

A *hip fusion* melds the pelvis and femur by removing the remaining cartilage and maintaining the two bones rigidly together until they heal to each other as would the two sides of a broken bone. No longer is there any mo-

> **Taking out the joint altogether can eliminate pain, but leaves the leg short.**

tion at the hip, the articulation having been fixed by the surgeon into one particular position. Pain is eliminated. There is only one problem: Everyday activities require the hip to move. The hip is straight when a person walks, and bent when a person sits or stoops to pick something up. If the hip is fused in the straight position (which is usually the case), sitting becomes very difficult. The person must sit at the very edge of any seat. Stairs are difficult.

A hip fusion might be recommended to someone who cannot undergo a hip replacement, such as a patient with a hip infection or someone who would subject his hip replacement to unusually high stresses (a construction worker, for example).

Resection arthroplasty is a fancy term for taking out the femoral head altogether. The empty space fills with scar tissue. This option is just as unpopular as the fusion for the opposite

> **Knee osteotomies are more common than their hip counterparts.**

reason: The leg isn't as stable as one would like it. The leg is also shortened by the procedure. Nevertheless, it can provide pain relief, and it is possible to walk with just the use of a cane and a shoe lift.

THE KNEE

Osteotomies are more frequently performed about the knee. The ideal candidate is young, heavy, and very physically active; he suffers from arthritis that is localized to just one side of the knee; and his tibia has a curve to it. In this situation, a cut is made in the bone and the patient is made more knock-kneed or more bowlegged depending on where the arthritis is located. If the arthritis is on the inside part of the knee (*medial*), the leg will be corrected to a more knock-kneed position to take stress off the arthritic side of the knee. Pain relief is not as predictable as with a total knee replacement, but as with a hip osteotomy, no special precautions need be taken by the patient once the osteotomy has healed. (Conversely, patients who have undergone a knee replacement are advised not to place heavy stresses across their knee for fear that the implant will loosen or wear out.)

There are many types of knee osteotomies: There are tibial osteotomies (just below the knee) and femoral osteotomies (just above the knee). There are closing osteotomies, whereby a wedge of bone is removed and the remaining edges of bone are brought together, and there are opening wedges, whereby a cut is made in the bone that is then opened. Your doctor's choice will depend on whom he's trained with, what he's read in journals, whom he's heard lecture, where he practices, and what his personal experience has been.

A bone that has undergone an osteotomy is unstable until it has healed. It, therefore, requires *fixation hardware,* a device that will secure the two sides of the bone. Such devices include casts, bone staples, plates, screws, and something called an external fixator—a TV antenna type of device that sticks out of the leg.

Because an osteotomy often takes a leg that is bending one way and bends it the other way, women are less likely to be pleased with the cosmetic results of an osteotomy than, say, a laborer who is mainly concerned with being able to go back to work.

The main complications of an osteotomy performed for arthritis include failure of the bone to heal (nonunion) and pain that persists even after the bone has healed. This presents the paradoxical scenario of an operation that has worked at the technical level but has nevertheless failed to provide the desired clinical result (pain relief). Such failures occur when the arthritis is simply too advanced or when the correction (the amount of bend the surgeon puts into the leg) has been insufficient. At the opposite extreme, *over*correction leads to a leg that looks excessively crooked. The surgeon sometimes treads a fine line between over- and undercorrection. Less common complications include injuries to the nerves and blood vessels surrounding the knee. Finally, an osteotomy can make an eventual knee replacement more technically challenging, especially in cases of overcorrection.

Chapter 4

What Exactly Is a Joint Replacement?

A joint replacement is a medical miracle whereby your joint is replaced with an artificial product. You may see the word *arthroplasty* here or there in your records. *Arthro-* means "joint" and -*plasty* means "alteration, reconstruction." Therefore, a hip replacement is sometimes referred to as a *hip arthroplasty. Total hip replacement* is abbreviated THR and *total hip arthroplasty* becomes THA.

> **Arthroplasty is another word for "joint replacement."**
> **A total hip replacement (THR), for example, can be called a total hip *arthroplasty* (THA).**

As discussed earlier, a joint consists of two bones coming together. The ends of the bone are covered with a white, glistening structure called *cartilage*, which allows the bones to quietly and painlessly glide about each other. Cartilage is eight times smoother than ice! When all is well, you move your knees, hips, shoulders, and fingers without giving them a second thought. But sometimes cartilage wears out. When it is completely worn down, and bare bone surfaces like the cement under a melting ice rink, motion in the joint is no longer smooth. In some patients this causes pain.

In joint replacement surgery the surgeon removes the worn-out surface and replaces or covers it with an artificial compound. This artificial structure can be made of any number of materials. These most commonly include metal alloys such as stainless steel, cobalt-chrome, and titanium products, as well as the plastic-like ultra-high molecular weight polyethylene (abbreviated with the easy-to-remember letters UHMWPE). But one also finds ceramic and, much less commonly, carbon.

> **The implant is either fixed to bone with orthopedic cement or is *press-fit*.**

HOW IS THE IMPLANT FIXED TO THE BONE?

Before we discuss the individual parts of a joint replacement, we need to talk about *fixation*, for it will help you understand some of the design concepts associated with the parts.

An implant has to be *fixed* to the bone, i.e., attached in such a way that it will not move at all. If it moves ever so slightly when you take a step, this will be painful. Because the forces imparted on your hip or knee replacement every time you take a step or get up from a chair are enormous, much work has gone into finding ways to fix your implant to the surrounding bone. Surgeons and engineers have come up with two solutions: An implant is fixed to bone by way of either orthopedic cement or by way of a technique called press-fit.

When the surgeon chooses cemented fixation, a white

paste is created by mixing a powder and a liquid. This paste (polymethylmethacrylate, aka PMMA) is introduced onto the surface of the bone, and the implant is placed against this paste-covered surface. In a matter of minutes the paste sets, i.e., hardens, and the implant is secure. You can pull or push on the implant and it will not budge. This orthopedic cement works in the same fashion as the cement between two bricks: it acts as a grout, filling in little interstices. Except in the early phase of setting, the cement is not sticky. It is *not* a glue.

> **Orthopedic cement is not glue. It is no stickier than cement in a brick wall, and it functions the same way.**

In a press-fit situation, the implant is wedged into the bone. The premise here is that the implant will be just a wee bit bigger than the bone and so will become jammed in. The surface of the implant has pores (tiny holes) into which it is hoped bone will grow. This process is called *bony ingrowth,* and it is this ingrown bone that over a period of months eventually secures the implant.

We'll address the pros and cons of each method later.

A HIP REPLACEMENT

As we saw in chapter 1, the hip joint consists of a round ball, the femoral head, and the matching concavity, the acetabulum. In a *total* joint replacement, both are operated upon. Classically, the femoral head is replaced by a ball perched on a *stem* (figure 4.1), and the acetabulum is resurfaced with a plastic or metal/plastic *cup* (figure 4.2). A number of variations on this theme exist.

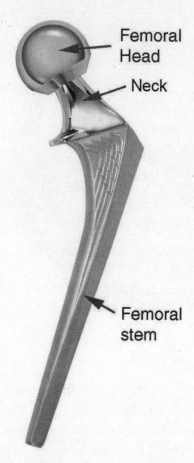

Femoral Head

Neck

Femoral stem

Figure 4.1 The stem and ball portion of a total hip replacement. (*Courtesy Stryker Howmedica Osteonics*)

The *stem and ball* can be made of one solid piece, or more commonly, the ball and stem are two separate components, in which case the implant is said to be *modular*. The part of the stem that protrudes from the bone consists of a tapered cone

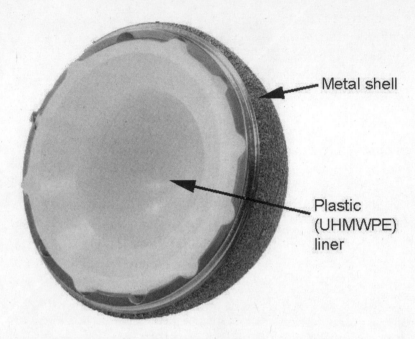

Figure 4.2 The cup portion of a total hip replacement. (*Courtesy DePuy Orthopaedics, Inc.*)

(a *Morse taper*), and the hollow ball (*head*) is literally tapped and wedged onto this Morse taper. The head is manufactured with a *neck* extension, and this neck extension varies in length. The surgeon chooses the neck length that gives the best fit. If the neck is too long, the surgeon won't be able to get the femoral head (ball) back into the cup, and/or the patient's leg will have been lengthened excessively (chapter 8). If the neck is too short, the construct is loosey-goosey, and the hip can pop out (dislocate) unexpectedly (see chapters 8 and 18).

The femoral head is made of metal or ceramic. The metal can be stainless steel, titanium, or cobalt-chrome. Titanium is rarely used because it is relatively soft and wears down (slowly) when it repeatedly rubs against the cup. Ceramics represent a large class of materials. They are smoother than any of the metals and lead to less friction and torque. A ceramic femoral head articulating against a ceramic cup, therefore, lasts longer than any other combination of materials used in hip replacement surgery. Certain ceramics, however, have been found to crack, and ceramics are expensive.

> **Implants are modular: They consist of two or more pieces that are assembled during the surgery and tailored to fit you.**

The diameter of the femoral head varies. Your own femoral head measures somewhere between 45 and 55 millimeters in diameter (about 2 inches). In a hip replacement, the head measures 22, 26, 28, or less commonly, 32 or 36 millimeters.

The reasons for this relate to principles in physics you learned in high school (unless you were out that day). And if you didn't care for physics then, I suggest you skip this paragraph. One of the complications of hip replacement surgery is loosening (see chapter 18). In time, the fixation of the implant to the bone can loosen and become painful. On the cup side of the implant, loosening is related to torque. Every time you take a step or, more significantly, get up from a chair, the femoral head (ball) applies a twisting moment (torque) to the cup. This torque is proportional to the diameter of the femoral head. The smaller the head diameter, the less the

> **In deciding what "femoral head" size to choose, your surgeon has to weigh a number of factors.**

torque, and the longer it will take for the cup to (painfully) loosen.

The size of the femoral head also influences the rate at which the plastic in the cup will wear out. The larger the head, the quicker the wear.

For all of these reasons, the inventor of hip replacement surgery, Sir John Charnley, chose a smallish 22-millimeter head size (22.25 millimeters, to be exact) for his pioneering hip replacement, the low friction arthroplasty, as he called it.

But there is another side to this femoral head business: Taken as an isolated parameter (which no surgeon should do), a small head size increases the risk of dislocation (see chapter 18), which occurs when the head "pops out" of the cup. This explains the existence of 26-, 28-, and 32-millimeter head sizes. The loosening and wear of plastic cups have been shown to be significantly increased with 32-millimeter heads, which explains why you are no longer likely to receive an implant with such a head size.

In short, the surgeon has the choice between a smaller head that will last longer but will be more prone to dislocation and a larger size that will not last as long but will be less prone to dislocate. The day loosening and wear are solved, you will see the reemergence of larger head sizes.

Picayune technical note: There are multiple possible causes of dislocation in any given patient. Factors relating to the hip implant itself include the diameter of the femoral head, the diameter of the neck (see figure 4.1), the *offset* of the stem (the distance from the center of the head to the long axis of the stem), and the depth of the femoral head within the cup.

A cemented stem is tapered. In other words, it is narrower at the bottom than at the top. When the stem is introduced into the viscous cement, the shape of the stem causes cement to be pressurized into the tiny cavities of the surrounding bone. These hundreds of little cement intrusions aid in the fixation. If the stem is of the press-fit variety, it may or may not be tapered. Here the surgeon's desire to use a tapered or non-tapered stem has to do with more complex issues of stress distribution, and these are beyond the scope of this book.

> **Press-fit stems are sometimes coated with a product that will enhance the growth of bone into the stem.**

The surface texture of a press-fit stem is usually rough. By presenting a sandpaper surface to the surrounding bone, it allows bone to grow into the tiny interstices of the implant surface. Engineers have worked out just how rough the sandpaper finish should be. Since the growth of bone into the implant is a biological and chemical process, it is hardly surprising to find that bone grows into certain surfaces better than it does into others. Bone grows particularly well into something called hydroxyapatite (HA), a white substance that coats certain implants. Such a coating is not essential. Bone also grows into titanium alloys, cobalt-chrome, and carbon.

The cup. Most cups in use today consist of a metal shell that is impacted into the pelvis. It is literally hammered into place with a mallet. A plastic cup called the *liner* is in turn impacted into this shell. In some models the metal shell is supplemented with sharp spikes or with screws to supplement the fixation. The plastic cup may or may not have a *lip,* a raised portion of the rim that contains the femoral head somewhat and makes it harder for the femoral head to pop out unexpectedly (dislocate).

The cup may be made entirely of plastic ("all-poly," in the orthopedic lingo), in which case it is cemented into place. Indeed, press-fit plastic cups have not worked well to date. Cemented all-poly cups are usually implanted in patients over the age of seventy but are also occasionally used in younger patients, especially if a press-fit cup does not fit as well as expected or if a large bone graft is going to be used and it is clear that very little bony ingrowth will take place (bone graft is dead bone and, therefore, cannot grow in and about the implant).

Unusual cups. In patients at particular risk for dislocation—patients who have already suffered a few dislocations, for example—a so-called *constrained* cup can be utilized. With this construct, the femoral head snaps into the cup and comes out with difficulty. Why is this not used in every case? The constraint increases the torque on the cup and increases the risk of loosening.

Certain models feature a ceramic liner. These are matched to a ceramic femoral head. The friction of ceramic on ceramic is lower than metal on plastic and lower even than ceramic on plastic. Cost, design considerations, and politics have limited the availability of these constructs.

All-metal cups have been reintroduced. Although they failed when first utilized in the 1950s, some investigators feel that new metallurgy will lead to success. The friction associated with a metal head rubbing on a metal cup would intuitively appear to be high. This is indeed what happened in the 1950s. But with today's designs and metals, the friction may, in fact, be lower than that seen between metal and plastic.

I believe that it is best to tailor the implant to the patient, and every surgeon would agree to this—at least in principle. In practice, some surgeons have used only one type of system and will not be comfortable with any other. For example, some orthopedic surgeons have never used a cemented cup and will use a cementless, press-fit cup regardless of the situation.

A KNEE REPLACEMENT

Whereas the hip joint consists of two bones (the pelvis and the thighbone), the knee joint has three bones: the thighbone (femur), the shinbone (tibia), and the kneecap (patella). The kneecap represents one more part that needs to be designed, one more source of pain.

> **The classic knee replacement resurfaces all three compartments of the knee.**

The Classic Knee Replacement

The classic knee replacement has three parts: the metallic cap that covers the end of the thighbone (femur), the plastic tray that covers the flat, top portion of the shinbone (tibia), and the plastic piece affixed to the underside of the kneecap (patella) (figure 4.3 a-d). In the last twenty years or so, the plastic covering the top of the shinbone has been placed onto a metallic tray, and it is this metallic tray that is fixed to the bone. More on that later.

> **Controversy persists as to when the kneecap needs to be resurfaced.**

The term *total knee replacement* isn't very good in my opinion because it conjures up the image of big chunks of bone being whacked out. In fact, only slivers of bone are removed. The end of the thighbone is

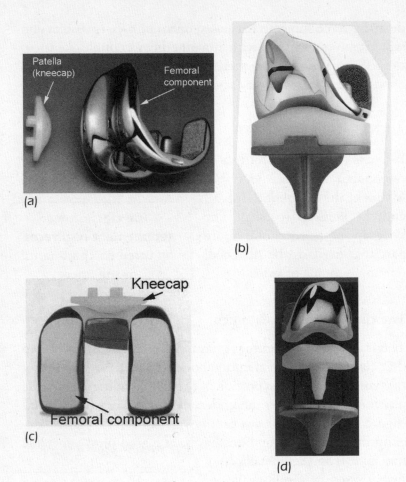

Figure 4.3 A total knee replacement. (a) the femoral head and patellar (kneecap) components (*Courtesy DePuy Orthopaedics, Inc.*) (b) the femoral and tibial component (*Courtesy Stryker Howmedica Osteonics*) (c) the patellar component as it fits onto the femoral component (*Courtesy DePuy Orthopaedics, Inc.*) (d) the tibial component disassembled into its plastic and metal parts (*Courtesy DePuy Orthopaedics, Inc.*)

shaped into connecting flat surfaces that will match a metallic cap. The upper shinbone is cut approximately at a right angle to its long axis, removing usually no more than a quarter inch of bone or so.

The kneecap is a hard bone with a very soft cartilaginous underbelly. This cartilage can wear out just like any other cartilage in the knee. In the classic knee replacement, the worn-out cartilage of the kneecap is removed along with a sliver of the underlying bone and is replaced by a plastic button (see figures 4.3a–d). The kneecap is then said to have been *resurfaced*.

As is the case with hip replacements, the implants can be fixed to the bone with cement or can be press-fit.

The Total Knee Replacement Without Kneecap Resurfacing

In this common variation, the kneecap is left alone, and just the thighbone and shinbone are operated on.

You should know that this is one of the major controversies in knee replacement surgery. Some surgeons feel that the kneecap should always be resurfaced, even if the cartilage appears only mildly worn. The reasoning here is that without resurfacing, the cartilage of the kneecap will be rubbing against the metallic implant covering the end of the thighbone. This can be a source of pain. Better to immediately place a plastic button under the kneecap.

> **The role of partial knee replacement remains one of the most controversial areas in all of orthopedics.**

The counterargument is that the kneecap portion of the replacement is a weak link in knee replacement surgery, being the one most likely cause of problems down the road. So why bother? It also adds time to the procedure.

Some studies seem to indicate that resurfacing the kneecap doesn't diminish the percentage of patients who have persistent pain after knee replacement surgery. This bolsters the argument for leaving the kneecap alone. But other studies point in the opposite direction, therefore the controversy.

In my practice, I went through a period of resurfacing every kneecap, then left a series of kneecaps unresurfaced, and now I leave the kneecap unresurfaced only if it looks healthy and my patient is unlikely to put much stress on the implant. I may change my mind again.

The Unicompartmental Knee Replacement

I take a deep breath here, for this subject opens a major Pandora's box. This is one of the most controversial areas in knee replacement surgery, a field already rife with controversies.

Let me briefly review certain features of knee anatomy (figure 13.1, page 161). There are three compartments in a knee, a situation analogous to an apartment with three rooms. The names of the compartments simply go by the two bones that make up that compartment. For example, on the inside part of the knee you have the *medial* (meaning "inside") *femorotibial* compartment. On the outside you find the *lateral* (meaning "outside") *femorotibial* compartment. The third compartment consists of the kneecap and the underlying thighbone and is, therefore, called the *patellofemoral* compartment.

Between the medial and lateral femorotibial compartments

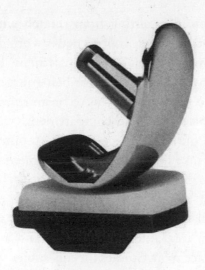

Figure 4.4 A partial (unicompartmental) knee replacement. (*Courtesy Smith and Nephew*)

lie the famous cruciate ligaments. Famous, or perhaps infamous, because anyone reading the sports pages has heard of the torn anterior cruciate ligament.

When only one compartment of the knee is arthritic, say the inside (medial) part of the knee, one can argue for just replacing that part of the knee and leaving the rest alone. It's not a new idea. It goes back to the earliest days of knee replacement surgery. Such a partial knee replacement is called a *unicompartmental* knee replacement, as it involves just one compartment of the knee (figure 4.4). It is abbreviated UKR and colloquially in orthopedic circles is called a "uni" (*u-nee*).

If a part in your car engine is broken, do you replace the part or do you change the whole engine? Obviously you change the part. But if a quarter to a third of the engine is broken, you may consider starting from scratch with a new engine. If only one compartment of a knee is worn down, do you limit the replacement to that one compartment? It depends on your point of view: Do you see this as being just one little part of the knee, or do you consider this to be an *entire* third of the knee? If you replace just one compartment, will the others eventually wear out, thus necessitating another operation? How long will it take for the other compartments to wear out? Is it possible that they will never wear out?

Faced with a patient with arthritis in one compartment (usually the medial, inner one), the orthopedic surgeon has a choice between a total knee replacement and a unicompartmental knee replacement. Studies on this subject support both points of view, and there exist an equal number of articles on both sides of the fence. In the United States, partial knee replacements have gone in and out of fashion over the last forty years. They tend to be more difficult than total knee replacements, yet surgeons are paid less (see chapter 20). Recently instruments have been developed allowing unicompartmental knee replacement to be carried out through a skin incision that is shorter than that of a total knee replacement, and interest in the procedure has been renewed.

I'm in the camp that believes that in carefully selected patients a unicompartmental replacement is good idea. I've been implanting them for over fifteen years. I'm not convinced that the overall recovery is always that much quicker (one of the purported advantages of a partial replacement), but patients do get home more quickly and they have an easier time moving their knee than their total knee replacement counterparts. If further surgery is ever needed, the surgeon has more bone left to work with than in a patient who has undergone a total knee replacement.

The Patellofemoral Replacement

An unusual variation on the unicompartmental replacement is the *patellofemoral* replacement, another procedure I've been a proponent of. Here the kneecap is resurfaced with a plastic button, and a metallic shield is placed in the *trochlear groove* of the thighbone. This procedure is reserved for patients whose arthritis is confined to the patellofemoral compartment, i.e., the kneecap and the underlying thighbone. The advantages and disadvantages of this replacement over the total knee replacement are similar to those discussed above in the section on unicompartmental replacements. There is less of a surgical dissection, the time spent in the hospital is shorter, the motion is better, but there is always the concern that another part of the knee might eventually wear out.

Such replacements have been available for the last twenty-five years, but much more so in Europe than in the United States. Reviews of this procedure have been mixed, as is the case for all unicompartmental replacements, and a surgeon can find any point of view backed up by at least one article in the literature. Most orthopedic surgeons have never seen this procedure and are not likely to offer it to you, but you should know that it exists.

Chapter 5

❖

Getting Ready for Surgery

Whether you are going in for hip or knee replacement surgery, the more you prepare, the smoother things will be. It's like everything else in life. And there are actually quite a number of items that you can and should address.

In the first place, you should educate yourself, which is what you are doing by reading this book. This has the effect of diminishing your anxiety and of giving you an element of control over your care.

GETTING IN SHAPE

You want to be in the best possible shape before your surgery. This includes your physical *and* your mental shape. As usual, the two are not completely unrelated. Being in good physical shape puts you in a good frame of mind, and a good attitude gives you the drive to address your physical shape.

You have to "think positive." You have to look forward to your operation; you want to have learned everything you can about your operation, your surgeon, and your hospital; and you want to go through the items listed below. You may want to meditate.

Exercise. Being in good physical shape can be difficult if you're in need of a hip or knee replacement! I recommend water exercises whenever possible. The buoyancy of the water allows you to perform activities that would be too painful or impossible on land. A light jog in the shallow end of the pool gets tiring very quickly. It's an excellent aerobic exercise and it'll strengthen multiple muscle groups about the hip and the knee. You don't even have to know how to swim and you don't have to get your head wet. One 45-minute session three days a week is a reasonable goal. The exercise regimen can be varied by running both forward and backward, and by performing limited jumping jacks. If there are two of you in the water, you can throw a Frisbee or a ball.

> It is important for you to *look forward* to your surgery.

Nutrition. Part of being in shape includes checking up on your nutrition. The better your nutritional status, the better your wound will heal and the lower your odds will be of developing an infection. "Of course my nutrition's okay. I eat all the time!" Well, it isn't so simple. It's not just a question of how much you eat, but also a question of *what* you eat—and what your body absorbs.

> It's not a question of how *much* you eat but how *well* you eat.

There are two blood tests that will give your doctor an idea of how well nourished you are. These measure the total lymphocyte count and the albu-

min level. Fortunately they are part of most routine blood testing protocols, and chances are that this information is already
in your doctor's chart. If not, these are easy, inexpensive tests
to obtain.

This nutritional information should be obtained as far in
advance as possible. Should the results suggest deficiencies,
there is time to modify your diet and time to repeat the test.

Stop Smoking.   Regardless of what type of anesthesia is
used, you will want your lungs to be as clear and clean as possible. This is because you will be on your back or on your side
for a prolonged period of time, and to a variable degree an area
of your lungs collapses on itself like a balloon deflating (a condition called *atelectasis*). This is a reversible condition, but in
the meantime it's a source of fever and weakness. You know
where I'm going with this: *Don't smoke!* The longer the smoke-
free interval prior to the surgery, the better.

Easy on the Drinking!   The other pleasure (or vice) that
can interfere with your recovery is alcohol. Nobody thinks of
himself or herself as being a heavy drinker. Nevertheless, you
should make sure your doctor knows how much alcohol you
drink, especially if it's more than wine with meals and the occasional drink. The more you drink, the less well nourished
you're likely to be (you're getting your calories from alcohol),
the less well your blood is going to coagulate, and in the severest cases you might go into DTs (delirium tremens) after surgery when your body is suddenly deprived of its daily alcohol.

Drinking irritates the lining of your stomach and predisposes you to gastritis and ulcers. This poses a problem because
after surgery you may be on a blood thinner (see chapters 10
and 15). Blood thinner plus stomach irritation equals bleeding
ulcer. Doesn't sound that bad? Try vomiting blood, passing

blood through your butt, or taking up residence in the Intensive Care Unit and see how that grabs you.

If you've been a heavy drinker, your liver hasn't been able to produce the normal clotting factors. You'll bleed more than normal during and after the surgery. This will make the surgery more difficult, you'll need more blood transfusions, and you'll be at increased risk for infection.

Bottom line: If you're a serious drinker, cut back dramatically on your drinking in the months before your surgery, and be sure to tell your surgeon how much you drink.

Your Teeth Need Attention! A little-known aspect of preoperative care is your dental health. Your mouth is one of the dirtiest parts of your body (bringing a different meaning to the term *foul mouth*). For example, a seemingly innocuous human bite wound that penetrates the skin over a knuckle earns the victim a trip to the operating room! A dog's mouth is less dirty! You don't want the bacteria in your mouth to travel down to your hip or knee replacement. This could cause an infection, always a serious event in a joint replacement. One of the causes of such bacterial migration is dental work. As the dentist rearranges your furniture, bacteria enter the bloodstream. By way of this bloodstream the bacteria travel through the body. At each stop your body fights them off. But around a joint replacement your body is at a disadvantage. Scar tissue doesn't have the normal immunological defenses, and bacteria can literally stick to the metal or to the plastic of your implant. The bacteria are free to grow and eventually you develop an infection. The way to minimize the risks of such an occurrence is to have any planned dental work *before* your joint replacement, ideally six weeks prior to the surgery—long enough to ensure the absence of a dental infection. This is particularly true if you already suffer from a dental abscess or infection.

Guys, Your Prostate Needs Attention Too.   Flat on your back, filled with pain medication, and recovering from anesthetics medications, you may find it hard to pee after your surgery. This is especially true if you had trouble before the surgery. This is the main reason for having prostate surgery before your joint replacement rather than afterward. The second reason is that your prostate surgery is a potential source of infection for your hip or knee implant. Any bacteria pushed into the bloodstream could land in your knee or hip and cause an infection for the reasons listed in the previous paragraph. Now don't get me wrong: I'm not suggesting that you have an unnecessary prostate operation. But *if* you're going to have prostate surgery, do so before your joint replacement. Speak to your urologist about this.

"Medical Clearance."   If you're really in the know, you don't use the term "medical clearance" anymore. The term "clearance" implies that your doctor guarantees you an absence of complications, which of course he or she cannot do. The modern term is "preoperative evaluation and management." The doctor checks that you are as well as you can be, tells you what your medical risks are, and advises the surgical and anesthetic team of extra medications that may need to be administered and of special precautions that may need to be taken.

> **Some insurance companies reimburse your family doctor very poorly for your preoperative evaluation, optimization, and "clearance."**

Joint replacement surgery is usually elective (you've peacefully picked the date in advance). Therefore, there is time to have your family doctor/internist give you the once-over. In fact, the anesthesiologist will demand this. This is the time to check up on any condition you've been nursing along, whether it be your blood pressure, your diabetes, your thyroid, etc. Your doctor may want a consultation with a vascular doctor, a cardiologist, or any other specialist. Make sure there's plenty of time to get this done, so don't wait until the last minute to see your doctor. The more medical conditions you have, the more time you want to give your doctor. In fact, you should contact your doctor as soon as a surgical date has been set. Your doctor's office may tell you that coming in a week before will suffice, but if there's any chance of your needing some extra testing, you should gently remind your doctor's staff that you suffer from or are at risk for such-and-such condition. When in doubt, get that extra consultation. No anesthesiologist has ever complained about too many consultations or tests. But an anesthesiologist will not hesitate to cancel your operation right there in the holding area if he or she feels that this or that condition has not been fully evaluated. Trust me on this one.

BLOOD DONATION

Blood management has been a "solution in evolution" for the last twenty years. The guidelines and recommendations are constantly changing.

We know that a certain amount of blood will be lost during and after your surgery.

How much blood loss can you tolerate? The specific answer to that is unknown. Generally speaking, the younger and healthier you are, the more blood loss you will tolerate. Conversely, the older and the more medical conditions you suffer from, the less your doctor will allow your blood count to drop before stepping in.

Once upon a time, you would receive a blood transfusion as soon as your blood count dropped below a magic number. Ahhhh, those were the days. Decision-making was easy. Now, in deciding whether or not to transfuse you, we evaluate your age, your health, the speed at which you seem to be losing blood, and how well you seem to be tolerating your low blood count. And whether you or your family has predonated blood. It's an imperfect science.

If your health is good enough, you will be given the option of donating your own blood prior to surgery. This is called pre-donation or *autologous donation* and is usually carried out at the hospital's blood bank. The blood bank stores the blood until the day you need it. If your blood count is high to begin with, your surgeon may decide that your odds of needing a transfusion will be too low to warrant this exercise. Conversely, if your blood count is on the low side to begin with, your doctor might not want to make you even more anemic by having you donate blood!

> **Fewer transfusions are administered today, but the decision-making has become more difficult.**

If it's been decided that you will predonate blood, this should be done about three weeks prior to surgery. Blood doesn't keep more than about a month. If the donation is carried out too close to the time of the operation, your body will not have had the time to replenish the blood that's been donated.

The advantage of predonating your blood is that you won't be getting a stranger's blood. But it's still not a guarantee. On rare occasions a clerical error is made and a patient gets the wrong blood. For this reason, even if you've predonated blood, your doctor may not order a transfusion unless he feels that you really need it.

Can my relatives and friends donate for me? Sure. First of all, that relative or friend needs to have the same blood types as you. Yes, types. The world of blood donation has gone way beyond the simple A, B, O matching. There are types, sub-types, and sub-subtypes. Your relative has to match you across the board. The blood bank also tests for viruses such as the HIV virus and various hepatitis viruses. And this brings up an interesting point. Your close relative can't always be counted on to fess up that he or she's been involved in activities that put him or her at risk for an HIV infection. Because of this, your relatives may be no safer than a total stranger. Consequently, blood banks no longer automatically encourage blood donation by relatives.

THE "VIRAL SCREEN"

If you harbor certain viruses, you put yourself and the operating room staff at risk. The two that come to mind are the hepatitis virus(es) and the HIV virus. You may be a carrier for these viruses and not even know it. In the case of the hepatitis C virus, a needle stick in the operating room can lead to the surgical or nursing team becoming infected. And the infection can be fatal, even if you yourself never had a day of symptoms! The HIV situation is more complicated. If the T-cell count is low and the viral load is high, you are at an increased risk of developing an infection after your joint replacement. And as with the hepatitis virus, the HIV virus can be transmitted to one or more members of the operating team. It may not even require something as dramatic as a needle stick. The virus can be aerosolized by the saws, reamers, and other orthopedic tools, and then breathed in by the operating team—at least theoretically. But HIV testing is not easy, and the surgeon may be discouraged from doing so. You can fight only so many battles.

> **Certain viruses may put you at an increased risk for an infection, while other viruses put the operating room staff at risk.**

PREPARING THE HOUSE

Presumably, you'll be coming back home at some point after your operation. Little preparations can make life easier. For example, if you have a shower stall, place handles on the wall. Throw rugs can be tripped over, so roll them up and put them aside until you are walking normally again. In fact, this is a good time to make sure there aren't telephone cords, computer cables, and the like that might pose a hazard. You don't have that much control over your existing pets, but this is not a good time to get a new cat or dog. They tend to walk right in front of you or even between your legs.

BEFORE THE SURGERY: A TIMELINE

Three weeks before surgery. Stop taking aspirin. If you take just a baby aspirin daily, it's acceptable to continue that, but double-check with your surgeon. Aspirin is a blood thinner. It works by modifying the function of your platelets, the clotting cells in your bloodstream. Since platelets live approximately three weeks, stopping aspirin three weeks before surgery assures you that none of your circulating platelets will have been compromised. Other anti-inflammatory medications such as Motrin, Advil, ibuprofen, Aleve, naproxen, Vioxx, and Celebrex can also affect platelet function, but not in such dramatic fashion. Stopping such medications just a few days before surgery suffices. Check with your doctor.

One week before surgery. As a last-minute check, the hospital will have you come in for basic tests. You will have the opportunity to see the hospital, check out transportation options to get there, and speak to an anesthesiologist. More on that below.

Switch to a low-residue diet a few days before surgery. Stay away from most fruits, vegetables, and nuts and focus more on meat and dairy (for once!). This will minimize your need for a bowel movement in the first day or two after surgery. In case your imagination hasn't filled in the blanks, here's why: First, the anesthetics and narcotics you will be receiving are terribly binding. Better that they not have much to bind. Second, getting out of bed isn't easy. If you have the urge to go one hour after you've just been put back to bed on the first day after surgery, the nurse might simply hand you a bedpan. Not the most pleasant option!

The day before surgery. By now, just about everything has been taken care of. You've read this book so you're an informed consumer and you are less anxious. You can eat and drink as much as you want, but only until midnight. After that you will be NPO, the abbreviation for the Latin version of "nothing by mouth." (Many medical terms come from the Greek and Latin. Once upon a time—and not all that long ago—Greek and Latin were mandatory subjects for medical students.) The reason for this is that the anesthesiologist will want your stomach to be empty. Aspiration pneumonia is a major complication that occurs when stomach contents go back up the esophagus and down the windpipe into a person's lungs. Stomach contents are extremely acidic. They can burn a hole in your skin, and that's exactly what they do to a pair of lungs. Normally food doesn't go back up the esophagus, but when you are anesthetized and lying down, it can happen. The best way to avoid this is to avoid having any food in your stomach altogether. If you figure that it takes eight hours for your stomach to empty and that the first surgery of the day takes place around 8 A.M., you'll understand why midnight is the cutoff time for both Cinderella and for you (and if you disobey, your lungs will turn to pumpkins and you will turn into a vegetable).

"But my surgery is not until two P.M. Why can't I have breakfast?" Good point. Theoretically, if you ate your breakfast at six A.M., you'd be all set for two P.M. The problem is that surgical schedules are not predictable. The case ahead of you might be canceled and you might need to be ready for eleven A.M.

> **You arrive at the hospital long before your surgery because there is much paperwork to be done and because surgical scheduling can be very imprecise.**

"But don't surgical schedules tend to run late, and won't I be famished by the late afternoon?" Good point again. But no doctor or hospital is going to have you eat breakfast because of that possible eventuality. Again, what if contrary to form, the operating room is running way ahead of schedule because of one or two cancellations? The hospital would look silly telling you that you couldn't be moved ahead because of their own recommendation that you eat breakfast!

"What about my morning medications?" That's exactly the question you want to ask the anesthesiologist when you visit him or her at preadmission testing (PAT). The anesthesiologist may have you take certain medications the morning of surgery with a sip of water. A sip of water. Not a tall glass of orange juice. A sip of water.

Having said that, you may brush your teeth (and floss). You may rinse your mouth and gargle to your heart's content, as long as nothing reaches your stomach.

Bathe. At the time of surgery your leg will be scrubbed with soap and painted with an antiseptic solution. Thus the dirtiest person can be "prepped" for surgery, but why take any chances? Start off clean!

PREADMISSION TESTING

A few days prior to the surgery you will be invited to the preadmission testing (PAT) area of the hospital. This is not an invitation you can turn down.

The visit serves multiple purposes. Simple blood tests are performed to double-check that your liver and kidneys are functioning adequately, that your sodium and potassium are normal, and that you are not anemic. These tests are often state-mandated. In other words, it's not your doctor or the hospital who demand these tests; it's the state. And the state demands that these tests be performed within a certain period of time, commonly a week, prior to the operation. Personally, I think it's a good idea. Your last blood tests may have been performed by your family doctor a few months earlier, and things can change. A cardiogram (EKG) and a chest X-ray (CXR) might also be performed depending on when you had them done last. A sample of your blood will be sent to the blood bank and analyzed. Should you need a blood transfusion (in excess of what has been predonated), the blood bank will already know your blood types.

> You might feel that preadmission testing at the hospital is a nuisance, but it's an opportunity to check out the hospital, examine parking and transportation, and speak to the anesthesiologist. It also ensures that your basic labs will be available the day of the surgery.

You may have the opportunity to speak to an anesthesiologist. This is the time to ask specific questions about general and spinal anesthesia. Bear in mind that the anesthesiologist may not commit to one type of anesthesia or another for fear of contradicting the anesthesiologist who will be taking care of you on the day of your surgery. As mentioned above, now is the time to discuss any medications or nutritional supplements you are taking, and what can and cannot be taken the morning of surgery.

On a more mundane level, going to PAT gives you an opportunity to check out the hospital. How are you going to get there? Where will you park? What is the nearest bus stop? Armed with that information, you will be less anxious on the day of the surgery.

Going to the hospital is a nuisance. Can't I have all these blood tests done by my family doctor? In theory, yes. Your doctor simply sends or faxes a copy of the blood tests to PAT and to your surgeon. That's the theory. In practice, your family doctor and his or her staff are busy. They may not have the fax number to PAT. They may wait until the last minute. The hospital gets anxious. Urgent phone calls are placed. Should the surgery be canceled??? You start doubting the competency of your doctors. For all of these reasons, I suggest you have the testing done in the PAT unit.

Besides which, if you don't go through PAT, the hospital may not allow you to have surgery in the morning. Delaying a morning case messes up the operating room schedule for the rest of the day, and hospitals have found that delays are much more likely to occur with patients who haven't been through the PAT process. And by now you know why. Patients are late arriving to the hospital because they underestimated their travel time, the cardiogram still hasn't arrived from the family doctor, etc.

THE DAY OF SURGERY/THE HOLDING AREA

You will need to be in the hospital long before your procedure starts.

You first get signed in, take off your street clothes, and get into a hospital gown. And wait.

When it looks as if they may soon be ready for you in the operating room, you go to the holding area, usually a large room just outside the operating suite. This is where the nurses look through your chart for the last time, making sure all is in order. You will speak to the anesthesiologist assigned to your operation, and the surgeon will have you sign the consent. In this consent you attest to the fact that you are not going into the operating room kicking and screaming against your will.

This form protects the surgeon and the hospital against charges of assault and battery.

Sometimes you sit or lie in the holding room for a very long time. This can be because the operation preceding yours is taking longer than expected. Or the staff assigned to cleaning your room are busy elsewhere. Or there's a change of shift. Or a piece of equipment needs to be sterilized. Even though there's often a television tuned in to the news, it's not unreasonable to bring a book or a magazine with you.

This "hurry up and wait" attitude on the part of the hospital can be irritating, but the hospital has to figure that some people will arrive late. Also you have to be all prepared and ready to go if the surgery preceding yours gets canceled.

> You will be pleased to know that hospitals are putting a maximal effort in eliminating wrong-sided surgery. You will be repeatedly asked what hip or knee is being operated on. While you are in the holding room, your surgeon may use indelible ink to mark the operative site.

You will be asked many times which leg is being operated on. This is to check, double-check and triple-check that no mistake is being made. In many hospitals a mark will be placed on the leg to be operated on. For example, your surgeon may place his initials near the planned surgical site. Wrong-sided surgery has been a major issue. It used to pop up regularly in the press. You wonder how such a thing could happen, but it's really not that hard. First of all, some people have a form of dyslexia that makes it hard for them to distinguish right from left. And some of these people are health professionals treating surgical patients! If you are on the operating table flat on your back with your knees draped over the end of the operating table, your right is to your nurse's left as she faces you. You may also be turned this way or that way for the surgery and this can compound the confusion.

In an ideal world the surgeon would be in the operating room while the skin is cleaned and the drapes are applied, but in reality he has commonly been called away to do something else or may be performing a procedure in another operating room. When he arrives, the leg has been cleaned ("prepped") and draped by the operating room staff. He may begin the operation without realizing that the procedure has been sabotaged. The solution to this problem is relatively simple: The surgeon places a mark in the planned operative site with an indelible marker, i.e., a mark that will not be washed away during the surgical prep. If he sees the mark on the skin, he knows that he's got the correct side. If not, he stops to review the situation.

A friend or relative can stay with you in the holding area. You can wear your glasses. The nurses will place your dentures in a cup and will ask you to remove any contact lenses. The anesthesiologist may choose to put in your intravenous (IV) line in the holding area, thus saving operating room time. There is usually a fair amount of hustle and bustle around you. Patients are coming in and out. Doctors and nurses are being paged overhead. There's usually a child crying. A pizza delivery guy might wander in. It's a happening place.

Part II

THE HIP

❖

Chapter 6

The History of
Hip Replacement Surgery

Hip arthritis has coexisted with man since his appearance on this planet. Men and women have resorted to herbal medications, canes, and wheelchairs to fight and compensate for this debilitating condition. They still do today. But in the nineteenth century, surgeons began to develop the tools necessary to treat this condition surgically, an effort that culminated in the 1960s with the development of the total hip replacement.

Left to its own devices, an arthritic hip will eventually stiffen up. This is the body's failed attempt at completely immobilizing the joint, a task that if successful would indeed eliminate pain. But since the human body is incompletely successful at immobilizing the hip, a person is simply left with a relatively stiff and painful joint. The first operations, therefore, consisted of providing the subject with more motion. White, Barton, and Sayres all performed a so-called osteotomy, whereby a cut is made in the bone. The cut was made below the stiff hip, thus creating a new joint of sorts. The patient's native joint was still present and painful, and though the osteotomy might have improved motion, it did little for the pain.

Another operation—the *resection arthroplasty*—simply removed the femoral head. It was popularized by Girdlestone and the concept is simple: If two bones are rubbing, remove one of them. The problem with the operation is obvious: If you remove the femoral head and replace it with nothing, the leg will be short. This effect can be minimized by placing the patient in traction after the surgery. The traction maintains open the space vacated by the femoral head, and within a few weeks scar tissue fills the void. The operation is still used today for patients who cannot undergo a total hip replacement and is colloquially called a "Girdlestone."

Fusing the hip presented yet another approach. In a *hip fusion* the femoral head is biologically welded to the pelvis. The surface of the femoral head and that of the acetabulum are roughened, and the hip is then immobilized by either a cast or a combination of orthopedic plates and screws. In time, the raw surfaces heal together as would two ends of a broken bone. A fused hip is indeed painless. However, the fusion doesn't always take, in which case motion between the bones persists and the patient still experiences pain. When the fusion works, the patient is left with a hip that doesn't hurt, but it doesn't bend. Sitting is difficult.

> **Prior to hip replacements, surgeons tried resection arthroplasties, fusions, and interposition arthroplasties.**

The next step in the development of hip arthritis surgery

consisted of an *interpositional arthroplasty.* The term *arthroplasty* refers to an operation that modifies an articulation, and the word *interpositional* refers to placing a tissue between the articulating surfaces of the hip joint. As we've seen, the hip joint resembles a ball in a socket, and in an interpositional arthroplasty, some tissue is placed between the ball and the socket. From the mid-1860s until the early 1950s, surgeons interposed every imaginable tissue, including muscles, skin, celluloid, silver plates, rubber, magnesium, zinc, and pig's bladder. All of this was done with the idea of reducing bone-to-bone friction and eliminating arthritic pain. Pig's bladder was actually quite popular at Johns Hopkins Hospital (presumably less so among Jewish and Muslim patients).

In the early 1920s, Smith-Petersen had the idea of fashioning a cap that would be placed over the arthritic femoral head to reduce friction. He first used glass, then moved on to Pyrex, Bakelite, and finally Vitallium cobalt-chrome, a metal already in use by dentists. This operation was called a *cup arthroplasty.*

Around the same time, surgeons thought of removing the femoral head altogether and replacing it with a ball-shaped device that would somehow be affixed to the rest of the femur. This left the door open for imaginative options. The ball was made of rubber, ivory, acrylic, and metal, and it was fixed to the femur by stems of variable lengths. One of the first popular hip replacements in the United States was a device called the Austin-Moore replacement (1953) and it was most commonly used in patients who'd suffered a certain type of hip fracture called a femoral neck fracture (see chapter 1). It consisted of a ball the size of the patient's femoral head and a smooth, dagger-like stem that went down the canal of the femur—one size fits all. Variations on the Austin-Moore included the Thompson (1950) and the Cathcart implants. For the elderly, low-demand, nursing home population, this worked reasonably well. But the "one size fits all" approach didn't work for the younger, more active population. The stem would often be loose within the femoral canal and cause pain. Moreover, if there was widespread arthritis present within the hip joint, removing the patient's femoral head and replacing it with an equal-sized metal ball just wasn't going to provide predictable pain relief. The metal ball rubbing against the arthritic acetabulum could still be painful. Surgeons needed a cup that could be affixed to the pelvis so the metal ball would have something other than the patient's own bone to rub against.

And that's where Sir John Charnley from Great Britain came into the picture. Actually, he wasn't a "Sir" yet. He was knighted later on for his contribution to joint replacement surgery. Although he did not invent the concept of the total hip replacement, he is credited with a number of innovations that turned the hip replacement from a frustrating dream to an everyday reality: After going through a number of iterations, he discovered a plastic that would be suitable as a cup. It wasn't easy, for an implantable material has to satisfy many requirements. It must not deteriorate in the highly corrosive, saline environment of the human body. It must not cause any damage to the host (patient). And if it's to last a patient's lifetime, it must be extremely durable. When a material satisfies these requirements, it is said to be *biocompatible*.

Charnley first tried Teflon but the tiny wear particles were extremely irritating to the tissues. Strike Teflon. Eventually he happened upon ultra-high molecular weight polyethylene

(UHMWPE), a material that is still in use today. In orthopedic lingo it is referred to as the "poly" (as in "What size poly are you putting in?"). Charnley also came up with the idea of fixing his implants to bone with a medical type of cement—polymethylmethacrylate (PMMA). Finally, after studying the mechanics of a hip replacement, he recognized that it would be advantageous for the femoral head

> **John Charnley was knighted in England for his development of the total hip replacement.**

at the top of his stem to be much smaller than a person's native femoral head. He came up with a head size of 22 millimeters. This metallic ball would articulate in a plastic cup that would have a 22-millimeter inner diameter. The cup and the stem would be affixed to bone with this PMMA. The era of joint replacement surgery was born. The Charnley hip is still in use today, and in patients over the age of seventy-five, no implant has proven to be better.

The Charnley hip wasn't perfect, however, and Charnley and his disciples tinkered with it. They altered the shape of the stem, for example. Eftekhar in New York devised the concept of creating numerous short drill holes in the cement to provide a better grip for the cement. Some of the big names in hip replacement surgery in the 1960s and 1970s also included Stinchfield at Columbia's New York Orthopaedic Hospital, Lazansky at the Hospital for Joint Diseases in New York, Harris and Aufranc in Boston, Amstutz in Los Angeles, as well as Wilson and his team at New York's Hospital for Special Surgery. Where Charnley operated on the hip by way of a so-called trochanteric osteotomy (a piece of the femoral bone is removed at the beginning of the operation and repositioned at the end), Müller in Switzerland implanted his replacements without such an osteotomy.

The hips that Charnley operated on would occasionally loosen, especially in younger patients. In joint replacement surgery, loosening generally leads to pain. New cementing techniques were developed: The femoral canal was washed with a water irrigation device similar to a Waterpik so that only solid, firm bone would be left for the cement to intrude into (the bone lining the inner aspect of the femoral canal is honeycombed— perfect for cement fixation). A plug was placed in the femoral canal a third or so of the way down. This kept the cement from being pushed to the bottom of the canal and, more importantly, allowed the cement to be "pressurized." Since the cement was blocked by the plug, as the surgeon introduced more cement, it was forced deeper into the walls of the canal. When the cement dried, this approach made for stronger fixation of the stem and less loosening. This technique, called second-generation cementing, is now widely utilized.

> **The traditional cemented hip replacement that works so well in older people works less well in the young. The younger the patient, the more the surgeon will try to do away with cement altogether.**

Less commonly used is *third-generation* cementing, whereby the cement is chilled (not stirred) and placed in a centrifuge to rid it of air bubbles. In the laboratory setting this makes for stronger cement, but it's not clear that it presents a benefit to the patient.

While improvements were being made in cement techniques, orthopedic surgeons also sought to do away with cement altogether. One approach developed through the 1980s involved coating the metallic implant with a rough surface. The implant would be forcefully yet carefully impacted into the bone, thus wedging the implant into position. The cementless implant was said to be *press-fit.* Bone would eventually grow into the tiny spaces provided by the rough surface. It took a great deal of trial and error to find an acceptable material and just the right surface roughness. Cobalt-chrome and titanium alloys were two products found to be acceptable, and they have both been widely used. In the late 1980s it also became acceptable to coat the implants with hydroxyapatite, a product that induces bone to grow into the implant.

Around 1985 another type of cementless cup caught on in the orthopedic community: screw-in cups. These cups featured threads that would literally be screwed into a patient's pelvis by way of large torque wrenches. They worked well for a few years, but a number of models suddenly loosened. In the end, the patients were screwed up in more ways than one.

Improvements in these cementless techniques have led many cups to be press-fit. The UHMWPE (poly) is placed within a metal shell, the outer aspect of which is rough and/or coated with hydroxyapatite. Some shells are peppered with holes through which screws are inserted. These screws sometimes provide even more solid fixation.

Through the 1970s, the metallic stems were made of one piece. This piece included the metallic ball at the top. This presented one major drawback. At the end of the operation, when the surgeon would "reduce" the hip (see chapter 8), there would sometimes be too much slack in the system. It would be too easy for the surgeon to place the femoral head into the cup, and this suggested that it would be easy for the patient to painfully dislocate their hip after surgery. In the 1980s, the orthopedic industry began to manufacture two-piece femoral implants (stems): the ball would now be a separate piece that would be snapped onto the stem. Attached to the ball would be a little protrusion called the neck. Sitting on a shelf in the operating room would be metallic balls with different neck lengths. Once the cup and the stem had been implanted, the surgeon could pick the ball with the best neck length. This type of stem is said to be *modular*. Modular stems are currently the norm. They do present a corrosion risk, however, and in select cases a surgeon might choose a one-piece stem (if he can find one).

Certain patients in need of a hip replacement suffer not from arthritis but from osteonecrosis (see chapter 1). In such a case, the problem lies entirely with the femoral head. The cartilage of the acetabulum is intact, at least initially. The concept was, therefore, developed from implanting a partial hip replacement for such patients. It would consist of the standard stem on top of which would sit the standard head (ball) measuring 22 to 28 millimeters across. A larger ball would snap on top of that ball. This larger ball would be lined with UHMWPE plastic on the inside and would be completely free to rotate both around the smaller ball and within the acetabulum. It was termed the *bipolar hip replacement*.

The operation was quicker than a total hip replacement because time was not expended preparing the acetabulum and inserting the cup. The rate of dislocation after surgery was much lower (see chapters 8 and 18) because of the large size of the ball. Finally, it was felt that if the cartilage of the acetabulum ever did wear out, the large metal ball could always be removed and a traditional cup could be inserted into the acetabulum. It was a clever idea and bipolar hip replacements remain widely available. The issue that has arisen is the following: If a patient is going to require a conversion from a bipolar to a total hip replacement within just a few years, would he not have been better off with a total hip replacement in the first place? Also the plastic inside the bipolar replacement can wear out just like the plastic portion of total hip replacement's cup.

Yes, like the brake pads in your car, the plastic portion of a total hip replacement can wear out. The obvious problem with plastic wear is that eventually the metal ball on top of the stem begins to rub against the metal shell behind the cup.

> **The weak link in a total hip replacement is the plastic bearing. Over time it gradually wears down—usually very, very slowly. The older the patient, the more likely it is to last a lifetime.**

This spells disaster because the hip joint fills up with metallic particles, and the metal shell that remains intact and well fixed to the bone must now be laboriously removed. A subtler problem goes by the term *osteolysis*. The microscopic particles of UHMWPE plastic that come from everyday wear elicit a biological reaction, the by-product of which results in bone loss. Imagine termites gradually eating away at the foundation of your house and you start to see the problem of osteolysis. So the less wear, the better. How quickly UHMWPE plastic wears out depends on the activity of the patient (the more you use it, the quicker it wears out), the specific implant (some designs are more fortuitous than others), and luck.

Yes, luck.

UHMWPE is not manufactured by orthopedic companies. It is an industrial product normally used in large blocks. Take two small pieces of any block and you'll find that they have differing mechanical properties. Thus two implants may wear out at very different rates. Could UHMWPE manufacturers make a more uniform product? It's not worth their effort. Orthopedic products make up just a tiny fraction of their business. In fact, UHMWPE manufacturers have gone in just the opposite direction: Some have stopped selling their product altogether to orthopedic companies. They're tired of being sued.

For the UHMWPE that is still being sold to us, numerous attempts have been made to make it more durable. Pull out any orthopedic journal from the mid-1980s and you will find advertisements for "carbon" UHMWPE. After intensive laboratory testing, the orthopedic companies released carbon-reinforced UHMWPE, a plastic that was going to be more uniform and more durable.

It was a bust.

Not only did it not last longer, but it wore out even more quickly than the original product and, to boot, left indelible charcoal black residue around the hip as far as the eye could see.

In the 1990s another company took a stab at the Holy Grail by processing UHMWPE in a way that would improve its longevity. Failure. They'd done plenty of laboratory testing, but never on *sterile* cups (why sterilize a piece of plastic sitting on a lab bench?). They consequently never realized that the new cups would be harmed by standard sterilization procedures. It may sound like an amusing oversight, but quite a number of patients have paid for all of these oversights.

A completely different approach is to do away with UHMWPE altogether. In the early 1970s surgeons in France began using ceramic. Ceramic is even smoother than metal. It, therefore, will cause less wear of the plastic (poly) with which it is articulating. The word *ceramic* actually encompasses a host of different products, and some have worked better than others. Some surgeons have been quick to dismiss ceramics because of

> **Ceramics have been a viable alternative to plastic, though they are expensive and haven't been problem-free.**

problems with one ceramic or another. Generally speaking, though, ceramics are prone to certain types of fractures and they are more challenging to manufacture than metallic implants. Their popularity and availability in the United States have waxed and waned.

At present some orthopedic surgeons are looking at other ways of doing away with the UHMWPE poly. In its latest incarnation, the metallic ball of the femoral component articulates directly with a metallic shell. This has already been tried in the past with poor results owing to the metal debris that is generated. The thinking, however, is that twenty-first-century machining can minimize the amount of metallic debris. Time will tell. Time will also tell whether even the small amount of debris will lead to long-term harm. Or not.

The latest fad (or is it an advance?) is the attempt to implant a total hip replacement through incisions so small that the surgeon can no longer directly see what he is doing. This inability to directly see the part of the body being operated on was the same criticism leveled at arthroscopists when they began operating on the knee by way of tiny incisions. In the case of the arthroscopists, however, their use of fiberoptic cameras was actually an improvement over what the naked eye can see. Not so here. Surgeons use crude, black-and-white X-rays for their minioperation and this is a poor substitute for the real thing. I predict a higher rate of complications with this approach, at least for the next few years.

Stay tuned for the second edition of this book to see whether this novelty has panned out or been panned.

Chapter 7

The Anatomy of the Hip

The *hip* is the name given to the junction of the thighbone and the pelvis. The hip is a joint, which means that it consists of two bones that are covered with cartilage and that articulate with each other. One side of the hip joint consists of the upper end of the thighbone (the *femur*), and on the other side you have a cavity in the pelvis called the *acetabulum* (figures 7.1 and 7.2). The word *acetabulum* has the same root as the Latin word for vinegar, acetic acid. Indeed some imaginative Roman anatomist must have felt that this portion of the hip joint looks like a vinegar cup. He was surely looking at an arthritic hip, for the normal acetabulum is shaped not like a cup but more like a horseshoe. It is the *arthritic* acetabulum that will sometimes be shaped like a cup.

The most prominent aspect of the upper femur is a round ball called the *femoral head*. This portion of the anatomy is frequently referred to throughout this book (figure 7.1).

The femoral head and the acetabulum are covered with *articular cartilage,* the white, smooth, shiny layer that allows for painless motion between bones.

The femoral head is connected to the rest of the femur by

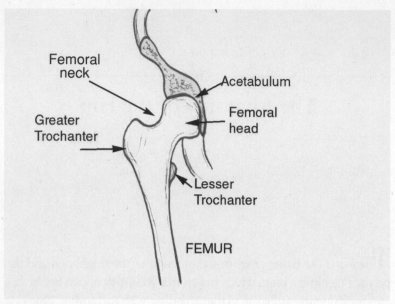

Figure 7.1 The hip is a "ball and socket" joint. The femur (thigh bone) articulates with the acetabulum (hip socket).

way of a relatively small, napkin ring–like segment called the *femoral neck* (figure 7.1). As we'll see later, a fracture of this femoral neck often leads to a hip replacement.

On the upper outer end of the femur there is a prominence called the *greater trochanter.* A little farther down, on the inner aspect of the femur, is a smaller prominence called the *lesser trochanter.* Hip fractures are classified according to their location relative to these two trochanters.

The hip joint allows for a remarkable amount of motion. Gymnasts and ballerinas can flex (bend) up to 180 degrees when they point the foot toward the ceiling or sit on the stage and rest their head on their shin. The hip can also be abducted

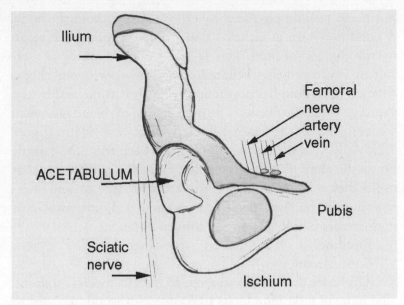

Figure 7.2 The pelvis and acetabulum.

(brought away from the midline) up to a right angle, as when the gymnast/ballerina performs a split. This terrific amount of motion is made possible by the ball and socket nature of the hip joint. The femoral head is the ball and the acetabulum is the socket. If you play with a skeletal model of the hip, you'll find that the leg can be placed in a wide variety of positions. In real life, the motion of the hip is limited by the ligaments connecting the femur to the pelvis. These ligaments exhibit a variable of stretch from patient to patient.

Like every joint, the hip is surrounded by tough tissue called the *capsule*. If fluid accumulates around the articulation, the capsule keeps it from leaking out. This fluid is most often normal joint fluid produced by every articulation in the body. A condition such as arthritis that irritates a joint leads to an overproduction of fluid. This is akin to tears forming as a result of your eye being irritated. Tears roll down your cheek, whereas joint fluid has nowhere to go as it is contained by the capsule. Occasionally, the fluid consists of blood as when someone breaks the femoral neck portion of their hip (figure 7.1). As long as the hip capsule has not been torn, the capsule limits the amount of bleeding that takes place. Fractures that occur below the capsule (the intertrochanteric and subtrochanteric fractures described in chapter 1) are associated with greater bleeding from the broken bone.

Bleeding?

Bone bleeds?

This came as a bit of a surprise to me as a medical student. The bone of a skeleton looks like a piece of wood; it's hard to imagine that it could bleed. Yet the situation is analogous to holding a starfish on the beach. It's dry, stiff, and solid. You can't imagine it as a supple living creature. Bone, however, is a living human tissue, thoroughly filled with arteries, veins, and blood. In fact, when a part of a bone loses its blood supply, the bone literally dies like the starfish pulled out of the sea.

The capsule surrounding the hip joint keeps the femoral head from rolling out of the acetabulum when you bend the hip to the extreme. Other structures that move the hip about and keep it in place are the muscles of the upper thigh. They completely surround the hip, front, back, and side. Although you can readily feel your knee under the skin, *you cannot feel your hip joint.* If you were unusually thin, you could feel it by pushing down in the groin area in the crease where the thigh joins the belly.

By and large, people suffering from pain that emanates from the hip have *groin pain*. People coming to the doctor's office rubbing their butt and complaining of "hip" pain are actually *unlikely* to have a hip problem. Their problem most likely comes from a pinched nerve in the lower back.

Chapter 8

✦✦✦

How Surgery Is Performed—
The "Routine" Hip Replacement

Most of you don't want to know. You've seen the procedure on television and that's enough.

But from my experience, some of you will appreciate knowing the technical details. So here we go.

When you enter the operating room, a nurse called the *circulating* nurse will greet you. Among many other things, he or she is in charge of getting you set up. You'll notice someone else who's not paying attention to you. This person already has their mask and sterile gown on, and that's the *scrub nurse*. This nurse will be handing the surgeon the necessary instruments during the operation. As you enter the operating room, the scrub nurse is busy setting up.

You'll note that the operating room is cool, perhaps frankly cold. That's because things warm up very quickly when the drapes are applied and the overhead operating lights are turned on. Also your surgeon will be wearing a gown and mask and it'll be a good 10 degrees warmer inside his suit. You don't want your surgeon and his team to be perspiring. If your surgeon is uncomfortable, he's more likely to want things to move along faster, which is not always to your advantage. Of equal significance is the issue of infection control. It is normal for people to shed bacteria through their clothing. Needless to say, you'd like to minimize this phenomenon near an open wound, and one way to do this is to minimize perspiration.

Prior to the start of the operation, you will be given a prophylactic antibiotic by way of your intravenous (IV) line. It's called prophylactic because it is administered prior to the onset of any infection. In fact, its job is not to cure but to prevent an infection. There has been more controversy with regard to this than you might imagine. In the 1970s it was felt that if a patient was given an antibiotic prior to

> **The operating room is cool. This is normal, and you will quickly warm up.**

surgery, he or she would simply become infected with a bacterium that was resistant to that antibiotic. Indeed, no antibiotic is effective against all bacteria. The surgeons who first administered these prophylactic antibiotics took a lot of heat from their colleagues. But lo and behold, the use of these antibiotics dropped the infection rate to less than 1 percent. The standard of care became to start the antibiotics before the surgery and continue them for five days thereafter ("post-op"). Surgeons cut this down to three days post-op, again taking flack from their colleagues. The current regimen consists of twenty-four hours of antibiotics with some investigators looking at just one dose before surgery. Sometimes today's malpractice is tomorrow's standard of care . . .

Choosing an antibiotic can be complex. The choice lies between an everyday broad-spectrum antibiotic that is likely to be effective against a number of common organisms versus the antibiotic most likely to be effective against the bacteria that are most prevalent in that particular hospital. The infectious diseases department of the hospital will assist with that decision.

Other than your surgeon, you may notice one or two other people scurrying around. These are your surgeon's assistants, and they are making sure that all the padding applied to your body to ensure that you won't get pressure sores is readily available. Pressure sores? Yes, you'll be lying in one position for a few hours and that's enough to develop pressure sores and related conditions, especially if you're on your side.

> **Once you're in the operating room, it takes time to get you set up. Anesthesia is carefully induced, a catheter may be passed into your bladder, you are positioned in a specific manner, and padding is applied to any possible pressure point.**

Anesthesia is administered in one of three ways: "general," spinal, or epidural. With general anesthesia, an intravenous medication puts you to sleep, and a plastic tube that has been gently slipped down your throat and connected to a little ventilator assures your breathing. Spinal and epidural anesthesia are closely related. A numbing medication is injected in your lower back, below the level of the spinal cord. The exact location of the tip of the needle determines whether the anesthetic is spinal or epidural. Either way, you are numb from the waist down. Intravenous medication makes you sleep during the operation, but it's not as deep a sleep as with general anesthesia, and you are breathing on your own. In the case of an epidural anesthetic, the anesthesiologist has the option of leaving a fine plastic catheter in your back through which pain medication can be administered for a day or two after the surgery. This seems like an ideal option except for the fact that the slightest displacement of the catheter makes the system ineffective. You will find a significant variation in enthusiasm for epidural anesthesia among anesthesiologists. Since post-operative pain is more of an issue after knee replacement surgery than after hip replacement surgery, the issue of an epidural anesthetic is more likely to come up if you are about to undergo a hip replacement.

Needless to say, there are pros and cons to each type of anesthetic. Factors to consider include your health, the medications you are taking, your back (spine) history, the experience of the anesthesiologist in any one particular area, of course, your personal apprehensions. At the time of your preadmission testing (see chapter 5) you can discuss this with an anesthesiologist.

A catheter may or may not be placed in your bladder. The standard varies from hospital to hospital. The advantage of such a catheter is that no one (including you) has to worry about whether you'll be able to pee after the operation. The combination of being flat on your back, receiving an anesthetic, and being administered pain medication can turn this routine act into an exercise in frustration. In long cases (and cases that take longer than expected), the catheter also keeps your bladder from becoming overly distended.

After anesthesia has been induced (that's the technical term for administering the medication that will make the operation pain-free), you are positioned on the operating table. Some surgeons prefer to perform the hip replacement with the subject lying on his or her back (the *supine* position), while others prefer the patient in the side position (*decubitus*). Either way, it is extremely important for the table to be flat and horizontal because the instruments used to insert the cup portion of the hip replacement reference off a flat, horizontal plane. If the table is tilted in one direction or the other, the cup may be improperly positioned. Some operating tables incorporate a button that automatically levels the table, but many do not. I always carry a carpenter's leveler just in case.

If the surgery is going to be performed with the patient lying on his or her side, time is expended to ensure that the person is "straight up and down." In other words, the patient has to lie exactly at 90 degrees to the horizontal. Again this is because the surgical instrumentation is designed on this premise. Ensuring that the patient is positioned correctly is not always as easy as it sounds. During the operation the leg will be moved this and that way, therefore tilting the patient's entire body one way or the other. It takes time and effort to secure the patient.

The leg is now "prepped." It is scrubbed to get any dirt off and then painted with alcohol and/or an iodine solution. Drapes are applied so that the only part of your body that is visible in the operating field is the leg to be operated on. Bright lights are focused onto the planned operative site.

While this is happening, a "cell-saver" machine is often set up. This sucks up blood that may ooze during the operation and saves it. The blood is then returned to you intravenously at the end of the surgery.

After making sure that "all systems are go," the surgeon

makes the incision. The exact shape and size of the incision depend on which approach the surgeon plans on using, the difficulty of the planned procedure, and the size of the patient's thigh. Hip incisions are usually well hidden by shorts, even short shorts.

You might have heard of tiny incisions being used for hip replacement surgery. These have the advantage of being even more cosmetic and perhaps there is less blood loss. But one of the keys to any operation is what surgeons call "exposure." You have to see what you're doing. If the surgeon's view is inadequate, you are at increased risk for a short- or long-term complication such as a dislocation, a fracture, or premature loosening of the implant. As with many innovations pertaining to joint replacement surgery, it can be not months but years before we know whether this new approach represents a step forward or backward (see chapter 19).

Having gone through skin, which is about the thickness of an orange peel, the surgeon then goes through a layer of fat.

> **Your friend has also undergone a hip replacement, but the skin incision seems different from yours. Indeed there exist a number of surgical approaches to the hip joint.**

Whereas men tend to have more fat around their belly, women accumulate fat around their upper thighs. It's the apple versus the pear. After the skin and the fat have been entered and parted, the surgeon has to decide which approach to take to get way down deep into the hip joint. Think of a house with many doors.

These approaches have names such as *anterior, posterior,*

Watson-Jones, trans-trochanteric, and *direct lateral.* By and large, the surgeon tries to part muscles as he might part a curtain rather than cut through them. In the direct lateral approach the surgeon goes through a muscle, but along its grain. The trans-trochanteric approach involves cutting the knobby part of the upper thighbone (you can feel it under your skin about a hand's breadth below the belt line). This knob is called the greater trochanter (a smaller knob on the inner aspect of the thighbone is called the lesser trochanter). The greater trochanter has a large muscle mass attached to it, and when you get it out of your way, the view that you have of the acetabulum and of the inside of the femur is unmatched by any other approach. The downside to this approach is that the greater trochanter has to be reattached at the end of the operation. This involves skills and complexities that add time to the operation, and they are not always considered by Medicare and insurance carriers as being worthy of any extra compensation (see chapter 20).

> To perform a hip replacement, the surgeon must pop the femoral head out of its socket. To this effect, he bends the hip and turns the leg inward.
>
> You do *not* want to do this inadvertently after surgery. This is a basic postoperative precaution.

Now that the surgeon can clearly see the large femoral head—the big round ball—inside the acetabulum, he's got to get this femoral head out so he can operate on it. This is called dislocating the hip. He cuts the thick layer of tissue that surrounds the whole joint called the capsule. The hip joint is bent past 90 degrees and slowly twisted inward. This usually

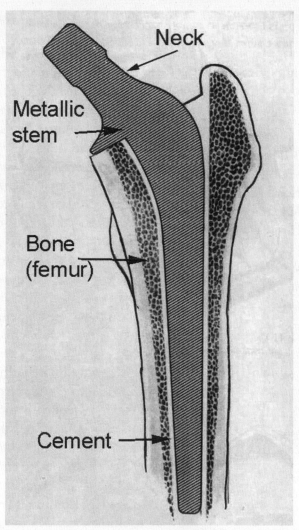

Figure 8.1. Cross-section of a cemented stem. The stem is fixed by the orthopedic cement that has worked its way into the honeycombed interstices of bone. The ball has not yet been impacted onto the neck of the implant. (*Courtesy DePuy Orthopaedics, Inc.*)

pops the hip out (which is why you don't want to do this after surgery!!!).

The femoral head is usually unhealthy—which is why you are having the surgery in the first place—and it is removed along with a portion of the "femoral neck" (see chapter 7). The femoral head and neck will be replaced by the hip replacement, which also has a head and neck (figure 8.1). Note that the replacement head and neck are smaller than the bone that has been removed (I review the biomechanical reasons for this in chapter 6).

> **Your surgeon will expend time ensuring that the cup is placed in its proper orientation.**
>
> **This will minimize (though not eliminate) the risk of a *dislocation* in the weeks, months, and years after surgery.**

The stem portion of the hip replacement will go down the hollow part of the thighbone. The head and neck will stick out. The head will fit snugly into the artificial cup, which will have been inserted into the pelvis.

The amount of bony neck that is removed is one of the determinants of how long your leg will be after surgery. If too small an amount is removed, the surgeon will have to pull on your leg to get the implant in and your leg will be lengthened. If a little too much is removed, there will be too much slack in the system and the hip will have a tendency to dislocate. The system can be fine-tuned later in the operation when the surgeon chooses the neck length of the implant.

> **The cement that is used for some implants is not glue. It is not sticky. It works as a grout, as does the cement in a brick wall.**

Having removed the diseased head and neck, the surgeon works toward getting good exposure of the acetabulum, the round depression in the pelvis that the femoral head used to fit into. Normally, the acetabulum is round. But in patients with arthritis it is not uncommonly oval or may even have some other, irregular shape. The surgeon now takes a *reamer* that looks like a round cheese-grater. Little by little he reams until the remaining cartilage has been removed and the cavity has become perfectly spherical. If the cup is going to be cemented into place, holes—anchor holes for the cement—are created throughout the bony bed of the acetabulum. The cement is prepared by mixing a powder with a liquid. A gooey paste, which at first is sticky, is thus created. This stickiness has led some to refer to the cement as glue, but this is an error. As the cement sets, it loses its sticky property. The cement is introduced into the acetabular cavity and pushed into those anchor holes in the bone. The plastic cup is now introduced into the cavity. The surgeon and his assistants remain still as the cement hardens.

Placing the cup in its correct orientation is a major concern to the surgeon. Incorrect placement of the cup is one of the causes of the dreaded complication of hip dislocation, whereby the femoral head (the round ball) pops out of the cup in a sudden and painful manner. But placing the cup in the correct orientation is not a perfect science, and judging the orientation of the cup after surgery by way of X-rays and scans is equally imperfect. Nevertheless, with careful positioning of the patient and of the operating table, the cup can be correctly positioned in the vast majority of cases.

If the cup is to be inserted without cement, each pass of the reamer has to be exactly along the same axis to maintain the acetabulum perfectly round. The cup is then literally banged into place (figure 8.2). It is said to be *press-fit*. There are no subtleties here except that the surgeon has to remain mindful of the orientation of the cup. The cup may have small spikes for added fixation into the bone, and in some cases the cup may even be affixed to the bone with screws. There are holes in these cups and the screws go right through the cup and into the surrounding bone. On the other side of the bone lie blood vessels and nerves, and the surgeon will take this into consideration as he selects the size and direction of the screws.

> **There is no harm in removing the marrow from the upper thighbone. This is *not* the marrow that manufactures the majority of your blood cells.**

The surgeon now turns his attention to the stem. The upper femur (thighbone) is somewhat hollow to begin with, but soft, mushy bone needs to be removed and the cavity (called the *canal*) needs to be shaped to accept the metallic stem.

Patients sometimes want to know whether it is harmful to remove the marrow from the bone since it is the marrow that creates the body's blood cells. No. Very few blood cells come from the marrow in the upper femur.

In order to prepare the upper femur to accept the implant, the leg has to be gently placed into a rather unnatural position—one that could not be duplicated by even the most loose-jointed person. This is the result of the surgeon having carefully peeled away some of the tissues surrounding the hip joint.

The surgeon resorts to special rasps called broaches to remove the loose bone from within the femoral canal. He may also use a power-driven reamer if the bone is too dense to be

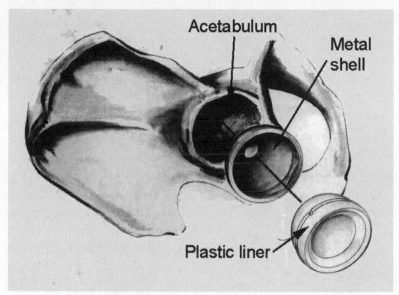

Figure 8.2. The cementless cup. The metallic shell is impacted into the bone and the plastic liner then impacted into the shell. (*Courtesy DePuy Orthopaedics, Inc.*)

shaped by hand. A trial stem is inserted into the canal. This gives the surgeon a chance to check the fit of the whole system before he's committed to the real thing.

Specifically, he places a round ball called the femoral head onto the trunion projecting up from the stem (called the neck of the implant) (see figures 8.1, 8.3, and 8.4). The leg is rotated back to its normal position and the orthopedic surgeon places the stem-femoral head combination into the cup. This is called *reducing* the hip. He now moves the leg in different directions to make sure that the femoral head doesn't slip out of the cup. If this were to happen after the surgery, it would be

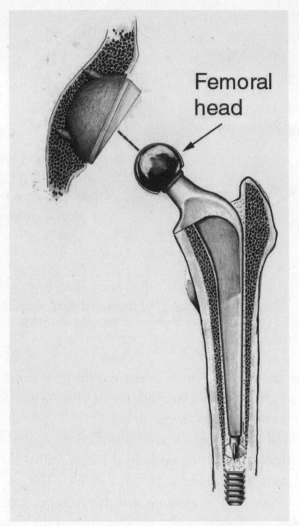

Femoral head

Figure 8.3. The final product. The round ball has been impacted onto the stem. Note the presence of a cementless cup fixed to the bone by three spikes (only two are visible here). (*Courtesy DePuy Orthopaedics, Inc.*)

called a dislocation. It is very painful. But it is not painful during the operation and the surgeon has an opportunity for fine-tuning before putting in the real implant. A hip is said to dislocate *anteriorly* if the head comes out toward the front of the thigh and *posteriorly* when it pops out toward the buttock. The less likely it is to pop out in one direction, the more likely it is to pop out in the other. The surgeon naturally tries to achieve reasonable stability in both directions.

> **Getting the leg lengths to match up is a concern to both the patient and the surgeon.**

The surgeon at this point also checks the length of the leg. *This is a tricky part of the operation.* The surgeon naturally wants both legs to be of equal length. If they were equal to begin with, he wants to maintain the status quo. If the operated leg was short, he will try to lengthen it. The difficulty comes from the fact that the hip is maintained in place ("reduced") by the tension of the muscles surrounding the hip joint. Think of the muscles as springs. As you stretch them, they become more taut. The longer the neck of the implant, the greater the tension on the muscles, and the greater their effectiveness in maintaining the hip's position. Parenthetically, this is why severe muscle weakness around the hip is a relative contraindication to hip replacement surgery. But the longer the neck of the implant, the longer the leg becomes. And therein lies the rub. The longer the neck, the stabler the hip, and the longer the leg. The surgeon each time around has to find the right compromise between hip stability and leg length. Sometimes the surgeon has no choice but to lengthen a patient's leg a fraction of an inch. If the leg was short to begin with, this usually presents no problem. But if the legs felt equal to the patient prior to the surgery, he or she may be displeased by the lengthening (see "Leg Length Discrepancies: A Further Discussion," page 118, for more on the subject). Hopefully this displeasure is offset by the marked pain relief they are now enjoying.

Once he is satisfied with the fit of the components, the surgeon implants the real stem. As with the cup, it will be either cemented or press-fit (figures 8.1, 8.3, and 8.4). Each has its advantages. A press-fit stem is hammered into the bone and there is a risk of fracturing it. Most cracks are small and of little clinical significance, but rarely, a major fracture will occur, and this will require a longer stem, plates, screws, etc. Most significantly, this leads to a lengthier operation and is, therefore, not a crowd pleaser. Press-fit ("cementless") stems, therefore, tend to be used in younger patients since their bone is less likely to fracture. Their main advantage is that they may last longer than cemented stems. Cemented stems have the reverse features. The femur is not at risk for fracture during the insertion of the stem. But the fixation of a cemented stem may not be as durable. Also note that press-fit, cementless stems and cups are significantly more expensive than their cemented counterparts (see chapter 20). In today's world the surgeon has to keep this in mind when deciding what system to use in a particular patient.

> **Cemented and press-fit implants both have certain advantages. Some surgeons routinely use just one or the other.**

With the stem in place, the surgeon proceeds to the last step of the operation. The real femoral head is impacted onto

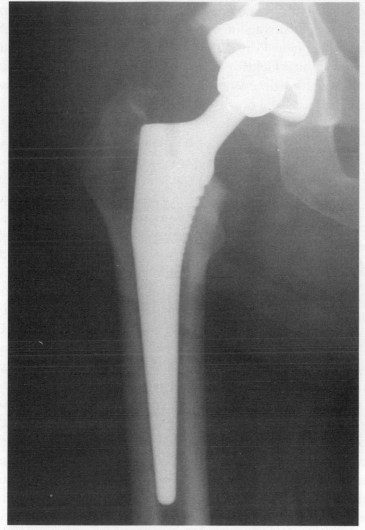

Figure 8.4 Cementless cup and stem.

the neck of the stem. The neck is slightly tapered (a "Morse taper" in engineering lingo). Once the head has been impacted (lightly hammered), it is impossible to pull off without the use of special instruments.

After this, the operation is essentially finished. The surgeon "reduces" the hip back together as he did with the trial implants. He again moves the hip systematically in different directions to ensure that it is stable.

> **Not long ago, a surgeon's failure to place a drain in the hip was grounds for malpractice. Now, many orthopedists consider drains to be irrelevant in routine hip operations.**

The wound is closed. Since many tissues about the hip joint were peeled away, not cut, the closure can be relatively quick. The main variable is the thickness of the fat layer under the skin.

Until a few years ago a drain would routinely be placed into the wound before the skin was closed. This was a plastic tube that was placed deep inside the joint and out the skin. The purpose of the drain was to prevent the accumulation of blood and fluid around the joint. Such fluid could seep through the skin for days on end and eventually could become infected. A surgeon could be sued for malpractice if he didn't use such a drain or if the drain slipped out prematurely. Now drains are considered useless, and some would say even dangerous since they theoretically allow bacteria from the outside world to enter the hip. Go figure. I use drains on cases that take longer than average to complete and remove them as quickly as possible. These days the use of drains is really up to the surgeon.

After a sterile dressing has been applied to the thigh, you are returned to the supine position (you're placed on your back). A large foam pillow may be placed between your legs to prevent you from moving your hip into a position that would put it at risk for a dislocation (e.g., bending the hip past 90 degrees and turning it à la cha-cha). Alternatively, you might find a brace wrapped around your knee. This may seem a little strange, maybe even a little scary. Did they operate on my knee??? No, it's not a mistake. If you can't bend the knee, then you're not going to be able to bend the hip past 90 degrees either! Try it.

An X-ray may be taken. If the stem was cemented, the X-ray will confirm that no major piece of cement leaked out unnoticed. It the stem was press-fit, the X-ray will verify that no major, unsuspected fracture occurred. These are unlikely scenarios, and the X-ray may not be taken until you get to the recovery room.

Once the anesthesiologist is satisfied with your condition, you are ready for the recovery room (occasionally called the PACU—pronounced *PAC-you*). But is the recovery room ready for you? Sometimes it's full! You wait in the operating room for a bed to free up. It's not too bad for you because you're groggy, but it's frustrating for your family (not to mention the next person waiting for their hip to be fixed).

How long you stay in the recovery room depends on how long it takes you to perk up from the operation—and whether your bed up on the orthopedic floor is ready. Your family will be eager to see you out of the recovery room, but the nurse-to-patient ratio is quite high in the recovery room and this translates to a great deal of attention. So personally I'm not in as much of a rush to see patients leave the recovery room.

LEG LENGTH DISCREPANCIES: A FURTHER DISCUSSION

Patients like to feel that their legs are of equal length, and every hip surgeon is aware of this. Once again, however, things are not as simple as they seem.

"True" Versus "Apparent" Leg Lengths

Patients want their leg lengths to be equal after surgery.

Actually, that's not completely true. They want their legs to *feel* equal.

The true leg length is the actual length of your leg: You place one end of a tape measure at the top of the thigh and the other end over the round bump on your ankle and this is a true measure of your leg length. If you take the same measurement on the other leg, you can now compare the two legs. If the measurements are the same, it is said that your true leg lengths are equal. But will they *feel* equal to you? Not necessarily.

> **There's a difference between your legs being of equal length and *feeling* equal.**

Your legs are connected to your pelvis. The round femoral head at the top of your thighbone fits into a round cavity on the side of your pelvis (the acetabulum). There's a right and left leg, therefore a right and left femoral head, and therefore a right and left acetabulum. If the pelvis is level, the right acetabulum and the left acetabulum lie at the same distance from the floor. In this situation, you will feel that your legs are of the same length.

However, if the pelvis is tilted—say the right side is higher—your right leg will feel short even though it is technically equal in length to the left. Try it. Stand up and hike up your right hip. Your right foot no longer touches the ground. If your pelvis were stuck in that position, you'd have to wear a lift under your right shoe. Yet your two legs are of equal length. If you were to apply a tape measure as described above, you'd still find the measurements to be equal on both sides. But place the top of the tape measure on your belly button and the other end of the tape on your ankles, and you'd find that the measurement on the right was shorter. This measurement is the *apparent* leg length and this is what you feel.

> **A tilted pelvis can alter your perception of leg length. So can tightness about the hip, knee, or ankle.**

The difference between the true and the apparent leg length that can exist when a "pelvic obliquity" exists is a potential source of confusion and miscommunication.

Take the example of Sally, whose right leg has always been short. The pelvis drops down on that side to compensate for it. Sally doesn't really notice that her pelvis is oblique and doesn't feel a difference in leg length. Her true leg lengths are different but the apparent leg lengths are equal. After a few decades the pelvic obliquity becomes fixed. Sally can't straighten out her pelvis even if she wants to. Suppose that Sally comes to a hip replacement. The surgeon removes the foreshortened hip and replaces it with a normal hip implant. The leg now is the equal of the other. Good job on the surgeon's part. But not so fast! Sally's pelvis still droops down on the operated side. And the obliquity is fixed. Sally can't bring the pelvis back to a level position. So the operated leg feels long!!! Sally isn't happy.

It can take a few months for a pelvis to adapt to a new leg length. You'll often hear surgeons recommend that patients wait two to three months before making permanent modifications to their shoe wear.

Are Leg Length Measurements Accurate?

Don't be shocked if different people get different readings when measuring your leg lengths. Your surgeon will tend to minimize the difference between your leg lengths. A health professional not interested in being friendly to your surgeon will maximize the difference. How is this possible?

> **A doctor not interested in being friendly to your surgeon can easily exaggerate the difference in your leg lengths.**

Measuring the length of a leg is not as simple as reading a number off a dial. You place a tape measure at one end of the leg and the other end of the tape at the ankle. Specifically, the doctor or therapist places the tape on the *medial malleolus*, the bump that sticks out above your shoe on the inner aspect of the ankle. This bump is broad and round. Depending on how tall you are, there can be a quarter-inch to a third of an inch leeway from the top to the bottom of that bump. At the other end, the measuring tape can be placed at the top, middle, or bottom of your belly button. Before you know it, one person says there's just a half-inch difference between your two legs and the other finds an inch of difference.

You would think that X-rays would be reasonably objective. Special X-rays can be ordered that image your entire leg. A ruler is placed next to the leg, and anybody can measure the distance from top to bottom. It isn't so easy. What if you bend your knee slightly? The leg will look shorter. No one looking at the films will notice this little artifact.

> **Many factors determine whether a person will or will not tolerate the difference in their leg lengths.**

How Much of a Leg Length Discrepancy Can You Tolerate?

It depends. The party line is that most patients will tolerate a difference of 1 centimeter or less (1 centimeter equals 0.39 inch). An inch or more will displease many patients, especially in routine cases. The exact level of tolerance depends a great deal on a person's level of expectation, on the demands of his or her lifestyle, on his or her appreciation of the surgeon's efforts, and on a person's tendency to see a glass as half full or half empty.

Interestingly, a person who's undergone a hip replacement for a hip fracture is more likely to be unhappy about a leg length discrepancy than someone who's undergone the same procedure for arthritis. See chapter 1 for a further discussion of this subject.

Chapter 9

❧

How Surgery Is Performed—
The Difficult Hip Replacement

In the previous chapter I reviewed the details of a routine hip replacement—if ever there is such a thing (I never approach an operation with the thought that it's going to be routine, though it often turns out to be).

> **Humans suffer from hip dysplasia too!**

Certain situations present special challenges. Fortunately the surgeon is often aware of these challenges prior to the surgery. He'll have allocated the extra time and have the necessary equipment.

HIP DYSPLASIA

You'll laugh if, like some of my friends, you've heard the term only in connection with dogs. But it happens not infrequently in humans. *Hip dysplasia* is the term given to a hip joint that doesn't have a normal shape. As we saw in chapter 7, the normal hip consists of a round ball (the *femoral head*) sitting in a round cavity (the *acetabulum*). The dysplastic hip differs from the normal hip in any number of ways—most commonly neither the femoral head nor the acetabulum is round. Their shape approximates an oval. The acetabulum is shallow, i.e., it looks more like a saucer than a cup. The front (*anterior*) wall is commonly deficient and this will lead the surgeon to give the cup an orientation slightly different from that of the routine hip replacement. The bone at the bottom of this kind of acetabulum is thick (this is actually helpful to the surgeon). The femur is skinny and the femoral canal (the semihollow portion at the center of the bone) is very narrow. The upper part of the femur might also be slightly twisted along its long axis.

The surgeon will need to convert the oval, shallow acetabulum into a spherical hollow deep enough to accept a metallic or plastic cup. Sometimes this requires a bone graft, a piece of bone that will be grafted onto your pelvis at the periphery of the acetabulum and then shaped. The graft is held in place by screws, and these are readily noted on an X-ray. Within a few months, the graft heals—becomes biologically connected—to the underlying bone and the screws are no longer necessary. Until the time when such healing occurs, you will need to walk with so-called protected weight-bearing. This means that the surgeon will not let you place all of your weight on the operated hip for fear that the graft will come loose. He will ask you to walk with crutches or a walker. The biological steps involved with the healing of the graft are complex and fascinating. After all, the graft is a dead piece of tissue. How does something inert become bonded to living bone? In short, the living tissue sends blood vessels and cells into the graft and gradually replaces it with living tissue. This is called "creeping substitution." It's a very slow process. Much work is currently being carried out on synthetic and semisynthetic graft materials that are "friendly" to bone ingrowth and generation.

On the femoral side, the surgeon may require an extranarrow stem and he may need to compensate for any femoral twisting ("rotation") he may come across.

In severer forms of dysplasia, the femoral head is not even resting in the acetabulum. This is called a *dislocated* hip. It's something one is born with. Pediatricians are attuned to this condition and usually test the hips soon after birth. Still, the physical examination is an imperfect science, and in some parts of the world testing isn't as rigorous as it should be. So some people slip through the cracks. They have a waddling gait, and upon obtaining an X-ray, they discover that their hip has been dislocated for all of their lives. This adds a layer of complexity to the operation. In a case like this, the surgeon will have to pull the femoral head down to the level of the acetabulum. It's not always so easy. There are blood vessels and nerves that are indirectly connected to the femur. These structures limit the amount of downward displacement that can be achieved, and conversely, pulling on the femur can injure nerves. The nerve most at risk is the sciatic nerve that runs down the back of the thigh. The sciatic nerve consists of two branches, one of which controls the ankle. This is the branch most likely to be affected by traction, and the result is called a *foot drop*. The patient can't lift the ankle. The ankle droops. The patient must, therefore, wear a plastic splint in his or her shoe to support the ankle.

Overall, though, you'll be glad to know that hip replacement surgery for hip dysplasia is generally successful. The operated leg is often short to begin with, and the surgery's natural tendency to lengthen the leg (see chapter 8) works to your advantage.

RHEUMATOID ARTHRITIS

Rheumatoid arthritis (RA) is a form of arthritis where the lining of the joint, the synovium, secretes a fluid that gradually wears out the cartilage covering the ends of the bone. When the condition exists from childhood, the condition is called juvenile rheumatoid arthritis and is abbreviated JRA. Patients with RA often take steroids such as prednisone. This medication has a number of wonderful features but one of its side effects is osteoporosis. Bones become thin and weak. The risk of fracture is, therefore, increased during a hip replacement. In patients with JRA, as with patients with a dysplastic hip, the femoral canal is occasionally found to be particularly narrow, necessitating special stems.

> **Patients of lesser education think it's called "sick as hell disease." It's not hard to imagine why.**

SICKLE CELL DISEASE

"Sick as hell disease" is how some patients pronounce this condition, and they aren't wrong. In addition to all the medical problems they suffer from, the bones around the hip joint can be made hard and marble-like as a result of this disorder. The hollow canal the stem is going to be inserted into can be completely obliterated by this hard, abnormal bone. The surgeon will have to create a new canal, a task that ranges from mildly challenging to brutally difficult and time-consuming.

Because the bone is not of normal quality, cement does not hold particularly well nor does bone grow normally into press-fit implants. This raises an entirely new set of problems.

Finally, patients with sickle cell disease are at increased risk for developing an infection about their joint replacement, a terrible complication even in the healthy patient.

But as of this writing, hip replacement surgery is still the best we have to offer sickle cell patients with hip disease, and many such patients have benefited from dramatic pain relief.

THE STIFF HIP

As we've seen, in order to remove the unhealthy, painful bone and replace it with an artificial implant, the surgeon needs to gently pull the hip joint apart. Specifically, he needs to pull the round "femoral head" out of the pelvic cavity called the acetabulum (see chapter 8). To do this, the leg and hip need to be relatively mobile. If not, the surgeon gradually releases the tissues that are holding him up until the femoral head can be teased out of its cavity. Occasionally, the femoral head feels like it is locked in. No matter how much tissue is peeled away, the hip does not budge, or not enough for it to come out. The surgeon must quickly switch to Plan B or C. That might include altering the sequence of the cuts, performing a trochanteric osteotomy (see chapter 8), etc.

PAGET'S DISEASE

If you are into medical trivia, you'll know what famous musician suffered greatly from one of the complications of Paget's disease.

Beethoven.

Paget's condition causes certain bones to become bowed and extremely dense. With Paget's disease the bones of the skull may grow to the point where a person's hat size will go up! Ever notice the prominent forehead on Beethoven's busts?

> **Which famous composer suffered from Paget's disease?**

But in Beethoven's case, that was the least of it. The growing skull can press on the acoustic nerves (the nerves connecting the ears to the brain).

Beethoven went deaf.

Had Beethoven undergone a hip replacement, his surgeon would not have been humming the "Ode to Joy." The canal into which the femoral stem is inserted can become obliterated as with sickle cell disease. It may also be bowed. The surgeon will see all of this on the X-ray. As a finishing touch, pagetoid bone can bleed considerably more than normal bone, all of which present significant obstacles to the surgeon.

POLIO

Patients with polio suffer from weakness of certain muscle groups. As I noted in the previous chapter, muscle tone is critical to keeping a hip replacement in place. Therefore, if a polio patient's diminished muscles surround a total hip replacement, they may not exert enough compression on the hip replacement to keep the hip in place. With polio patients the hip is at risk for dislocating. In such a situation the patient may require a special cup or the leg may need to be lengthened more than usual to create enough muscle tension.

THE REVISION (REDO) SURGERY

"So what if my hip or knee wears out? You'll just put in another one." Hmmmmm. Here's why this is not a good way to look at things.

> Revision (redo) joint replacement surgery is often successful. However, it is a longer and riskier procedure than the first time around.

When part or all of a hip replacement is redone, this is called a *revision* hip replacement. This can be a formidable procedure. "The surgery of surprise," I've always called it. It might be quite easy and straightforward—but it can also bring the surgeon to his knees. There are three parts to a revision: the implant is removed, bone deficiencies are addressed, and the new parts are inserted. Each of these presents special challenges.

Removing the Implant

First, you have to get to it. In the last chapter I described the surgical approaches to the hip joint, i.e., how the surgeon gets down to the hipbones. The surgeon has the same choice of approaches during a revision. With one major difference: The tissues are no longer soft and pliable. They are tough and leathery as a result of the first surgery. There is a great deal of scar tissue. This tissue is white or beige, it hugs the bone, and fills every cavity. This tenacious scar tissue has to be removed bit by bit so the surgeon can move the leg into the right position. If the surgeon tries to move the leg before enough scar tissue has been removed, the femur can crack. Did I mention the fact that scar tissue can be vascular? Well, it isn't really. But the surgical dissection required to remove all this scar tissue can lead to bleeding. The surgeon is working in a "wet" field. And no, it's not possible to use a tourniquet during hip surgery as you can when replacing a knee.

The surgeon "dislocates" the hip. This is what he'd been working so hard to keep you from doing on your own before the surgery. The femoral head is disengaged from the cup. The surgeon is looking right into the cup and directly at the top of the round femoral head.

What happens next depends on which portion(s) of the implant need to be removed. By and large the parts that are working well are left in place, and the surgeon will focus on removing the parts of the implant that need replacing. However, the parts may not cooperate. They may be quite well fixed to the bone. Even implants said to be "loose" can be in there pretty tightly. "Loose" is a very relative term. Imagine trying to take a brick out of a wall without damaging any of the surrounding bricks. The surgeon faces a similar challenge in taking out an implant without damaging the surrounding bone. It's very tedious and the clock is ticking.

Filling In Bone Defects

The surgeon is not working with normal bone. In some areas it will have become very thin. The gritty, honeycombed layer lining the bone will have disappeared, leaving behind an inhospitable, marble-like surface. Some bone may be altogether missing. The presence of bone defects and the quality of the remaining bone will determine to a large extent the difficulty of the operation. Sometimes these factors can be determined during the preoperative planning. But sometimes there are surprises. And surgeons tend not to like surprises.

If bone is missing, the surgeon has a number of options. If a defect is small, he can ignore it. Larger defects need to be replaced. The surgeon will take a large piece of bone from a bone bank (either cadaveric bone or bone removed at the time of someone's hip replacement) and fashion it to fit the defect. On occasion the bone will be ground down to a paste and then placed into a cavity. Many types of synthetic bone grafts are available but long-term results of these synthetics are not available.

Less commonly, the surgeon will make use of a so-called cage, in particular when there exist one or more major defects. If a surgeon tells you that he is considering a cage, you know that he's dealing with a tough technical problem. A cage is a metallic shell shaped like a normal acetabulum. Attached to this shell are little wings and flat hooks. These wings and hooks have holes through which screws can be inserted and fastened to what's left of the surrounding pelvis. A plastic cup is then cemented into the cage. There are gaps between the cage and the surrounding pelvis, and these gaps will have been filled with some form of graft prior to the insertion of the plastic cup. The surgeon hopes that the graft "takes" (heals to your bone) before the screws and cage work themselves loose. It can be a close race.

Your surgeon will juggle a number of factors in deciding what's best for you: the size of the defect(s), the location of the defect(s), the number of defects, your size, your age, your health, the availability of bone grafts, and the availability of (expensive) synthetics. As a rule, the bigger, younger, and healthier you are, the more he's going to be willing to let the clock tick away as he reconstructs your hip. Conversely, if you are older and less healthy, he's going to pay more attention to getting you off the operating table in a timely fashion. As usual, it's a judgment call on the part of the surgeon.

Introducing the New Implant

An implant has to be fixed to the bone. Either it is fixed with orthopedic cement or it is press-fit (jammed) into the bone. As we've seen, the cement works just like the cement between two bricks. It insinuates itself into the hundreds of little cavities present at the surface of the two bricks, and when it's set, the two bricks are locked together. The cement is not sticky. It is not a glue. In a "virgin" hip replacement (called *primary*), the surface of the bone isn't perfectly smooth. The hard, wood-like "cortical" bone is covered with a gritty type of bone featuring thousands of little nooks and crannies. This type of bone is perfect for accepting cement. In a revision situation, that gritty bone unfortunately is no longer present. What's left is smooth bone with no interstices for cement to enter. Therefore, if the surgeon is going to use cement, he will first have to roughen up that glassy surface. The press-fit situation is not much easier. Bone has to grow up to and into the implant if it's going to remain well fixed over time. That hard, marble-like bone may be alive but it's a poor source of bone-creating cells. On the femoral side of the hip, the surgeon will choose to use a longer stem than the one originally implanted. At least the lower part of the implant will be in contact with untouched bone. On the acetabular (pelvis) side the surgeon will use a cheese grater–like device to get down to what is referred to as "bleeding bone," bone that will provide cells for growth of new bone.

In a primary (nonrevision) hip replacement, the surgeon makes use of a trial implant in the femur. He then reduces the hip (see chapter 8) and verifies the stability of the hip (does the hip pop out with the leg in a certain position?). In a revision situation it is not always possible to use a trial for the femur. The trial may fit too loosely to give an accurate measure of what will happen when the real stem is implanted. The surgeon goes with his instinct and experience.

The complications associated with revision surgery are the same as those found with any hip replacement surgery. But the odds of suffering from one of these complications are greater.

Because the operation is longer, there is a greater chance of infection, and because the surgical dissection is greater, there is more blood loss and a greater need for blood transfusions.

Finally, because the tissues do not have their usual elasticity, because the surgeon may have been limited in his ability to place the implants just where he would have liked to, and because he may not have benefited from a trial reduction, the risks of your suffering from a dislocation are greater. This last risk accounts for the fact that your surgeon may place you in a "hip spica" brace (also called "hip abduction" brace). You are not likely to welcome it: Although it's relatively lightweight (compared to the cast it has replaced), it nevertheless still wraps around the waist and continues on down the thigh on the side of the operation. It doesn't let you move the hip very much, which means that it is difficult to sit down. Sitting in a car, in a chair, or even on the toilet is a chore. It is unsightly since it must be worn over your clothes. However, there is an alternative. We are currently developing a pad that fits *under* your clothing and doesn't wrap around your waist. It still limits your ability to bend the hip (that is, after all, the purpose of these braces and pads) but it does so in a cosmetic, user-friendly fashion.

The bottom line? Take good care of your hip replacement. Avoid running, jumping, and twisting. Treat it as though you could never have another one.

Chapter 10

Your Hospital Stay, Day by Day

Your recovery will be smoother and less filled with anxiety if you know exactly what to expect on a day-by-day basis. Note that the following outline may vary from hospital to hospital.

THE DAY OF SURGERY

On the day of surgery, not much is expected of you. Enjoy the rest. You'll spend a few hours in the recovery room, after which you will be transferred to your room. Regardless of the type of anesthesia, you will be groggy. The nurses will check your blood count and your vital signs, i.e., your blood pressure, temperature, pulse, and respirations. They will also check your level of pain, sometimes called the fifth vital sign.

If you have a catheter (called a Foley) in your bladder, they will monitor your urine output as a measure of how well hydrated you are, and if the surgeon has placed a drain around your hip joint, they will assess how much blood is being drained away.

Your family will be allowed to visit you in the recovery room. In some recovery rooms only one person at a time is allowed in. Note that in certain hospitals the recovery room is called the PACU (Post-Anesthesia Care Unit).

POSTOPERATIVE DAY 1

Out of bed. That's the catchphrase of your first postoperative day. Be prepared not to be in the mood to do so. You may even feel that they are rushing you. But it's important on many fronts: Your sense of well-being will be enhanced, your breathing will improve, your muscles will be put to use, you won't develop bedsores, you're less likely to get a rash on your back, and it will be easier to eat or drink.

> **The nurses and physical therapists will be getting you out of bed rather quickly!**

You won't walk much this first day, but the physical therapist will at least have you standing up.

You won't be very hungry, but it will be important for you to at least start taking in fluids.

If you've had a Foley catheter placed in your bladder or a drain about the hip incision, there's a good chance they'll be coming out. Although the catheter is convenient to the extent that you don't need to use a urinal or bed pan, its presence increases the risk of a urinary tract infection, which could in turn spread to your fresh hip operation.

The hip drain also presents a risk of infection. Until the 1990s, hip drains were considered critical. They were left in place until the amount of drainage dropped below a magic number. If the drain came out accidentally in the recovery room, that was reason enough to take the patient back to the operating room. Now drains are considered superfluous much of the time. It just goes to show how quickly the standard of care can change.

If you're not taking in much by mouth because you're not feeling well, the IV (intravenous) line will stay in your arm and provide you with fluid and basic salt.

You'll be encouraged to perform simple bed exercises. These are designed to keep the blood circulating (as opposed to pooling in your legs), to keep your muscles fresh, and to keep your lungs well expanded. Such exercises include ankle pumps, whereby you pump the ankles back and forth as if you were pushing up and down on a gas pedal, and inhaling and exhaling exercises using a plastic incentive spirometer.

There may be a frame attached to your bed, and hanging from that frame in the neighborhood of your chest you may find a large triangle called a trapeze. This trapeze is a device that you grab when you want to lift yourself off the bed. Lifting yourself up and letting yourself back down is a good exercise.

Your pain medication will be administered by way of injections or by way of your IV. Usually you have to ask for pain medication. It's not administered automatically. The reason for this is that your doctor doesn't want you to receive a narcotic that you don't need. The downside to this, of course, is that nurses rarely appear the moment you call for them. My advice is to ask for pain medication as soon as you think you might need it. You are usually allowed an injection every three hours.

PCA stands for patient-controlled anesthesia. In some hospitals your pain medication will be placed in a pump, and when you press a button, a small amount of pain medication flows into your vein. You press the button whenever you feel the need for pain medication. Of course, the anesthesia pain team controls how much medication is delivered with each push of the button and how many "deliveries" can take place in a given period of time.

Alternate ways of administering pain medication include epidural catheters, nerve blocks (injections), and skin patches. An epidural catheter is a soft, plastic tube placed in your lower back at the time of surgery. It can be left in place after surgery, in which case an anesthetic solution is continuously allowed to drip into the epidural space. This space is near the spinal cord. A numbing medication in this area blocks the pain fibers to the legs and provides pain relief. Because the epidural space is small, the anesthesiologist may not be able to place the tip of the catheter directly into that space. Even if the catheter is perfectly placed, it may wiggle out of position after surgery when you get out of bed.

> **You will be happy to know that pain control has become a major priority. It is now considered the "fifth vital sign" (following pulse, respiration, blood pressure, and heart rate).**

One of the risks of hip replacement surgery is dislocation, whereby the hip ball pops out of the socket (see chapters 11 and 18). Right away the staff will start to discuss with you the steps to take to avoid such a complication, mainly avoiding hip flexion past 90 degrees. In English, that means not bending your hip past a right angle. It also helps to keep your leg "abducted," in other words, away from the other leg (the opposite of crossing your legs).

You may still be groggy and unable to fully cooperate. You

will, therefore, find your legs attached to a big foam pillow that keeps you from bending the hip altogether. Less punitive is the "knee immobilizer," a contraption wrapped around the operated legs and fixed with Velcro straps. Nurses who are unfamiliar with hip replacement surgery will wonder why you are sporting a *knee* brace when you've had hip surgery. The reason is simple: Patients who can't bend their *knee* aren't going to bend their *hip* very far either (unless they are particularly loose-jointed). Try it.

> **Learning the basic precautions for preventing a hip dislocation is extremely important.**

Although it is essential for blood to clot, clotting in the wrong place and at the wrong time is potentially troublesome. Patients shudder at the term *blood clot,* and although they don't exactly know why, they are correct to be concerned. Patients who undergo hip replacement surgery are at risk for developing clots in the deep veins of the leg. This condition is called (deep) phlebitis or deep vein thrombosis and is abbreviated DVT. At best you don't feel it and it is harmless. At worse, a large clot floats up through your heart and into your lung, causing a *pulmonary embolus.* This can leave you very short of breath and in extreme cases can be fatal. A number of approaches have been tried to minimize this risk. They include tablets such as warfarin and aspirin, injections of a low-molecular heparin (such as Lovenox, Fragmin, and Arixtra), calf pumps, and ankle pumps, to name only the most common ones. Although all of these decrease the risk of phlebitis, it's not clear at all that they diminish the overall risk of death. Nevertheless, diminishing the risk of phlebitis is a good thing, and you'll probably find yourself receiving one of these treatments. Your calves, thighs, and/or feet may be wrapped in devices that inflate on a regular basis and squeeze your leg.

Blood will be drawn from your arm and sent for analysis. This will determine your blood count, i.e., it will tell the doctor the extent to which you are anemic (a certain amount of anemia is normal after a hip replacement). Your doctor may also choose to check your potassium, sodium, and other so-called chemistries.

You can expect a temperature of up to 101 degrees that may persist up to a week.

POSTOPERATIVE DAY 2

What a difference a day makes. By now you're much more with it. You'll want to know from your surgeon how the operation went and you'll want to be more active. You may even have some of your appetite back. You'll pretty much be free of tubes. And yet, you're still not yourself. You may still require shots for pain or still want the use of your PCA pump.

Today you start walking for real. The surgeon will have left instructions with respect to how much weight you can put on your operated leg, and the physical therapist will coach you in the use of a walker or crutches. How long you will need these devices depends partly on your specific type of hip replacement and partly on your surgeon's philosophy.

You will be encouraged to start taking pain medication by way of tablets in view of ridding you of catheters and needles.

Your diet will progress to solid food if you tolerate it. If you're on a special diet, the hospital will usually be able to accommodate you. I encourage relatives to bring in a patient's favorite food. After all, poor food is how a hospital gets you out!!! Soups and shakes go down easily. No, alcohol is not allowed. But this does bring up an important point. If you're a heavy drinker, you could go into DTs (delirium tremens). It's important to let your doctors know ahead of time if you drink more than socially. And by the way, going into DTs is not a way to get your hands on a drink: you'll be treated with a sedative, not vodka.

> **Pain diminishes dramatically every day.**

You will still be encouraged to perform the bed exercises you were shown on Postoperative Day 1.

The staff will again review the hip dislocation precautions. They are very important, so if the instructions aren't clear, make sure that the staff explains them again differently until you are satisfied.

The timing of the first dressing change varies from hospital to hospital. It is most commonly performed on Postoperative Day 2, 3, or 4. It's not a very convenient endeavor. The dressing is on your upper thigh and buttock, which means that you are going to have to roll over onto your other side to expose the whole dressing. This dressing change will be performed by a physicians' assistant, nurse practitioner, or resident (a resident is a surgeon training to become an orthopedic surgeon). A much smaller dressing will now be applied to your incision.

Blood will again be drawn to check your level of anemia. It can take a few days for your blood count to level off. If you are on a blood thinner called Coumadin (the brand name for warfarin), a test called the INR and a test called a pro time are performed on your blood sample to check the extent to which your blood has been thinned. It can take quite a few days to find just the right dose for you. It's a tricky situation because an insufficient dose might leave you unprotected against clots while an excessive dose can lead you to bleed excessively. But the margin between one extreme and the other can be very narrow, and the medication takes two days to work. So today's blood test assesses the effect of the warfarin dose from two days ago! You can see why warfarin is not very popular. But if you are going to need a blood thinner for a few weeks or months, it's still one of the more popular options.

POSTOPERATIVE DAY 3

You are now free of tubes. Under supervision you will start to get out of bed by yourself. The hip dislocation precautions will be reviewed with you. This is your opportunity to double-check that they've been explained and demonstrated to your satisfaction.

You will start to walk up and down the hallway. There may be some pain, but it will be very different from your preoperative pain: you will note surgical soreness, as opposed to the grinding, lancing pain you experienced before.

At this point your pain medication will consist of pills, freeing you up from IVs and injections.

The anticoagulation measures will still be in effect, as they will be during your whole hospital stay.

Depending on the hospital setting, you might be able to shower.

Expect swelling in the operated leg. It does not mean that you have developed blood clots. In fact, the correlation between blood clots and leg swelling is poor. For this reason, your surgeon may choose to automatically obtain a "duplex" test that examines your leg for clots. These duplex tests are kinder, gentler versions of a venogram, whereby dye is injected into a vein. A duplex test is painless.

Your team will be checking the amount of liquid drainage present on your dressing. It should taper off on a daily basis.

If you are cleared by physical therapy and if the drainage from your wound has essentially ceased, you might be discharged from the hospital later in the day or tomorrow morning.

POSTOPERATIVE DAY 4

If you were still somewhat groggy or unsteady on Day 3, or if your wound still exhibited significant drainage, your surgeon will keep you in the hospital. The presence of drainage may or may not lead your surgeon to put you back on antibiotics. This is a controversial area.

The routine will be the same: getting out of bed, walking, learning to become more independent, anticoagulation . . .

POSTOPERATIVE DAY 5

This is another potential day of discharge. You will need clearance from the physical therapist, and your wound will need to be essentially dry.

Persistent drainage can eventually lead to an infection, and your surgeon may choose to take you back to the operating room to wash out the hip *before* it becomes infected.

AFTER THE HOSPITAL

When you leave the hospital, you will either go home or be transferred to an inpatient rehabilitation facility. This rehabilitation unit might be in a hospital (such as the one you are already in) or in a nursing home (skilled nursing facility).

Either way, you want to be clear on the plans, precautions, and danger signs. The plans will include follow-up with your doctor, therapy you are supposed to receive, and medications you are supposed to take. The precautions will include the dislocation precautions that have already been drummed into you. They will also include infection precautions (see chapter 18). Danger signs include a temperature of 101 degrees or greater a week or more after the surgery, increasing redness about the incision, increasing swelling (remember: some swelling is normal), increasing pain, and any kind of drainage. Some health professionals are not aware of the risks posed by persistent oozing. They are falsely reassured by the fact that the drainage consists of clear liquid and doesn't appear to be infected.

You should go home with some basic equipment—or at least obtain it very soon upon arriving home. This includes a grabber to help you pick objects off the floor and a raised toilet seat. Devices also exist to assist you with putting on socks.

Your surgeon may want you to continue wearing the knee immobilizer to keep you from overbending your hip.

Chapter 11

Going Home After
Hip Replacement Surgery

Gee, it's good to be back home. The hospital wasn't so bad after all, but it's nice to be home. If nothing else, it's good to be in your own bed and not be disturbed by all those hospital noises. Heck, get up when you feel like it.

The good news is that not much is required on your part at this time. The operated tissues simply need time to heal.

EXERCISING AFTER HIP REPLACEMENT SURGERY

The muscles about the hip do not take much of a beating during the average hip replacement. By and large, the surgeon has parted the muscles rather than cut through them.

Nevertheless, the hip is bruised and this in itself will temporarily weaken the leg. This can be addressed by way of exercise. Exercises are divided into two categories: strengthening and functional training.

The term *strengthening* is self-explanatory. As you use your muscles, they become stronger. The key to any strengthening program is, therefore, to work your muscles a little harder than what they've been used to, and this usually means lifting or pushing a weight. Your leg makes for a pretty good weight, and so a basic hip exercise is to lie on your back and raise your leg,

> **Exercising is divided into strengthening and functional training.**

count to 10, and let it down. This is called straight leg raising. The first time around, you won't be able to hold the leg up for 10 seconds. Do what you can and progressively work up to 10 seconds. *Caution:* This can stress your back. If you are prone to back pain or sciatica (a pinched nerve down the leg), back off on this exercise at the first hint of pain.

Straight leg raising strengthens the muscles at the front of the hip and thigh. There exist, of course, muscles all about the hip and thigh and these also require strengthening. The muscles on the outside of the hip are called the *abductors*. Abduction means pulling the leg away from the body, and the ultimate example of abduction is a dog lifting its leg against a fire hydrant. The abductor muscles keep your pelvis level when you walk. Without the abductors of your *right* hip, you would fall to the *left* every time you took a step with your left foot. If it sounds confusing, don't worry. Even medical students scratch their heads on this one. For now, you'll just take my word for it when I tell you that strengthening your abductors is important. Fortunately, strengthening the abductors is easy: You lie on your unoperated side and lift the operated leg in the air. Count to 10 and let it down. This is just another form of straight leg raising. And equally boring. I recommend watching television or listening to music while performing these exercises.

Caution: After certain surgical approaches to the hip, including the trochanteric osteotomy (see chapter 8), your surgeon will want you to hold off on exercising the abductors for up to twelve weeks after your surgery. This is because your abductor muscles are attached to a part of the thighbone called the greater trochanter. If the greater trochanter has been detached and then reattached with some form of wire fixation, forceful contraction of the abductor muscles could work the wire loose. The surgeon may want the muscles about the hip to remain quiet until the trochanter has healed back to the femur.

> **If the surgery has been performed by way of a trochanteric osteotomy, your surgeon may want you to hold off on certain exercises for up to twelve weeks.**

The adductor muscles run along the inside of the thigh and they work to pull the leg toward the opposite leg. You bring your legs together by activating the adductor muscles of each leg. Strengthening these muscles is not quite as practical, but fortunately these have been relatively unaffected by the surgery. They lie on the inner thigh, opposite to where your surgery took place. To strengthen the muscles, push your legs together and count to 10. Alternatively, if you can place a heavy bag between your legs (for example, a bag filled with copies of this book), use the operated leg to push the bag toward the other leg.

The muscles at the back of the hip include the gluteus maximus, the muscle that creates the outline of your buttock. Strengthening this muscle requires lying on your stomach and lifting the leg. This will cause your back to arch. If it is painful, stop.

Functional training means that you simulate activities that are important to you. Walking, for example. The best way to simulate walking is, well, to walk. Not only do you strengthen your muscles, but you retrain them to work in concert. The analogy to music is appropriate: All members of an orchestra must work with seamless precision to produce a harmonious sound, and all muscles about the leg must work with equal harmony to produce a smooth gait.

> **Walking in the shallow end of a swimming pool is an outstanding exercise.**

If you have access to a swimming pool, walking in the shallow end is an outstanding exercise. Because you are buoyant, you place little stress across the operated hip, and the resistance of the water provides a reasonable challenge to the hip and thigh muscles. For variety, try walking backward and sideways. You may also use a kickboard or swim. Both the freestyle and the breast stroke are acceptable.

DRIVING, SEX, ETC.

One of the major complications following hip replacement surgery is hip dislocation (see chapters 8, 10, and 18), and many of your surgeon's admonitions will be geared toward avoiding this painful event. In particular, your surgeon will want you to avoid bending your hip past a right angle, especially if your leg is *adducted*, i.e., pointing toward the other leg. During the six- to twelve-week healing period, a thick layer of tissue forms around the hip joint. This tissue to a certain extent helps keep the hip joint in place. Your surgeon may, therefore, be somewhat more liberal with the activities he permits once this healing period is over.

When you pose the question "Can I do this?" the surgeon will think of the position you'll be putting your hip in during that activity. Driving can be problematic for a tall person in a low-lying seat, since the hip is nearly automatically bent past a right angle. You may want to place a cushion on the seat and, of course, keep the leg abducted. Ask the physical therapist to go over this with you. Depending on your size, the type of car you drive, and your surgeon's overall philosophy, you may be restricted from driving for up to twelve weeks.

The same considerations apply to sex. If your hip is not flexed past a right angle and your leg is not adducted, sexual activity poses no risk. The missionary position is safe for women and men. In fact, this is the safest position for a woman. For a man, the woman-on-top position is the safest. The "doggie" position is safe for the person who is upright. Pain and tenderness about the operated hip remain the limiting factors for any sexual activity.

Note: The advice listed in this section on driving and sex applies to patients who have undergone a traditional (in the United States) posterior approach to the hip. With other surgical approaches, bending of the hip is not an issue, but full straightening of the hip might be! Driving may pose no problem and neither would sexual positions in which the hip is bent to a right angle.

Each surgical approach has its pros and cons, and your surgeon will most certainly let you know which surgical approach was used and what activities need to be avoided.

HOME PRECAUTIONS

Hopefully, you'll have gotten your home ready *prior* to the surgery, but it's not too late to do so now. To avoid a dislocation, your surgeon will most likely want you to shower rather than sit in a tub. A bath mat and wall handles are a good idea since a shower tends to be a slippery place. Your foot can get caught in throw rugs, and your balance isn't back to normal, so have the rugs removed. Don't walk in the dark. Turn on a light if you must get up at night, and you'll avoid tripping on that shoe.

Part III

THE KNEE

Chapter 12

The History of
Knee Replacement Surgery

We take knee replacement surgery for granted, a testament to how far the world of orthopedic surgery has come. But knee replacements have been with us for only about thirty years. What did your parents, grandparents, and ancestors do? For the most part, nothing. At least nothing surgical. Surgery for knee arthritis was a creation of the twentieth century.

In many ways, the development of knee surgery mirrored that of the hip. Surgeons first attempted *interpositional arthroplasties*. An arthroplasty, by way of reminder, is an operation that reconstructs a joint (*arthro-*, "joint"; *-plasty*, "reconstruction"). In an interpositional reconstruction, the surgeon interposes a structure between the two worn-out surfaces of bone that are rubbing against each other. Surgeons experimented with just about every soft tissue that exists within a mammalian body, including pig's bladder. It didn't work. The interposed tissues quickly wore out.

As with the hip, surgeons *fused* the bones of the knee together. This certainly took care of the pain, but the stiff knee proved to be as unpopular as the stiff hip.

Encouraged by the results of cup arthroplasties in the hip, surgeons created a metallic cap for the far end of the femur. It didn't work either. MacIntosh in 1958 developed the concept of a small acrylic chip that would be inserted between the femur and the tibia. McKeever developed a similar implant made of metal. The first leap into the world of joint replacement surgery as we understand it today was made by Gunston in the late 1960s. Borrowing a page from Sir John Charnley (see chapter 6), Gunston used polymethylmethacrylate (PMMA) cement to fix two metallic runners along the end of the femur that would articulate with two pieces of UHMWPE plastic, themselves fixed to the tibia with PMMA. Thus, his total knee replacement consisted of four separate pieces.

It was only natural that someone would think of connecting the two metallic runners on the femur and the two plastic trays on the tibia. The Duo Condylar implant finally connected the two femoral runners. Freeman, one of the pioneers in the area of knee replacements, produced an implant that featured a one-piece metallic femoral component and a one-piece plastic tibial component. Insall, another pioneer in knee replacement surgery, designed the Total Condylar Prosthesis, which also consisted of one metallic cap on the femur and one plastic tray on the tibia. His other innovation was to remove worn-out cartilage from under the kneecap and replace it with a hemispherical plastic button. Interestingly, Insall and Freeman were both from Great Britain.

Most of today's total knee replacements are similar in appearance to Insall's original Total Condylar Prosthesis.

Some models feature a prominence in the middle of the plastic tray. These implants are termed *posterior stabilized* and are designed to allow the patient more bending at the knee. The importance of such a prominence is subject to debate.

As with their cousins, the hip replacements, knee replacements became *modular*. The plastic tibial tray became a two-part implant, consisting of a metal tray into which the plastic would be inserted. The metal tray was cemented into the bone as was the femoral component, and as the last step of the surgery, the surgeon would snap in the plastic, having chosen just the right size at the last moment. This eliminated the problem of cementing in all the components only to find that the plastic really should have been a little thicker or thinner. Any implant you receive today is likely to be modular. This is no longer a subject of controversy.

> **Modularity has been a true advance. The surgeon can fine-tune the fit of the construct until the last minute.**

A major advance took place in the late 1970s when Buechel and Pappas popularized the concept of a *rotating platform*. The plastic tray was free to swivel within the metal tray. This addressed a concept that is somewhat subtle: As the knee bends and straightens, the femur and tibia (thighbone and shinbone) rotate relative to one another. If, as you sit, you straighten your knee, your tibia will rotate outward. Conversely, when you bend the knee, it will rotate inward. You can't feel this happening, and you have to look closely at your leg to notice it. This repeated torque can cause an implant to loosen or wear. The rotating plastic follows the femur and swivels on the metal tray. The metal tray, therefore, doesn't "see" the torque and is less likely to loosen. A rotating platform allows for other design benefits, and a major opponent of this approach, knee pioneer John Insall, was testing his own rotating platform design when he passed away.

The components of a knee replacement have traditionally been fixed to the bone with PMMA cement. As was the case with hips, however, surgeons in the 1980s sought to fasten a knee replacement to the bone without resorting to cement. This gave rise to press-fit implants, which were pressed into the bone, the idea being that bone would grow into the small interstices at the surface of the implant. Some implants included screws for additional stability. However, whereas cementless hip replacements became more popular (especially the "cup" portion), cementless knee replacements have (temporarily?) fallen out of favor. They simply haven't been found to improve the clinical results.

> How long should a knee replacement last? If it makes it past the first two years, a number of models will last you more than twenty years.

So how long should a knee replacement last?

In a small number of patients, the implant loosens early on. The specific cause sometimes remains a mystery. A low-grade infection or a metal allergy can potentially lead to early failure of the replacement, yet be difficult or impossible to diagnose with certainty. If the replacement was implanted without cement, it is possible that a small amount of motion between the replacement and the bone prevented the construct from ever taking.

Barring such occurrences, a total knee replacement can last over twenty years. Perhaps much more. The models currently in use haven't been around much over twenty years. In fact, most models have existed for far less time. The limiting factor is often the plastic, which wears over time. The wear debris in turn causes bone to fritter away and the implant to loosen. The extent to which this happens varies dramatically from implant to implant and therefore from patient to patient. For this reason, to the extent possible I try to use implants with a long, successful track record.

PARTIAL KNEE REPLACEMENTS, AKA UNICOMPARTMENTAL REPLACEMENTS

Anatomically, the knee can be likened to an apartment with three rooms. The three rooms are called compartments. If just one compartment is arthritic, why replace all three? Thus the concept of the unicompartmental replacement. It consists of a small metal piece covering one condyle of the femur (see chapter 14) articulating with a plastic tray that sits on top of the tibia. This implant was popularized by Marmor from California in the 1970s. It has remained a staple of knee replacement surgery, its popularity waxing and waning throughout the years. Instruments have recently been introduced allowing for the implantation of unicompartmental replacements through incisions smaller than those of a total knee replacement and this has contributed to a renewed interest in the subject. By and large, patients sporting a unicompartmental replacement can bend the knee farther back than if they had a total knee replacement. On the other hand, because two out of three knee compartments remain untouched, there remains the chance that one or both of the other compartments will eventually be affected by osteoarthritis. Note that unicompartmental replacements are technically more than simply half a total knee replacement, being in some ways more complex than their larger cousins, and not all knee surgeons are philosophically or surgically comfortable with their use.

In the late 1970s, another set of Californians, Bechtol and Blazina, gave us the *patellofemoral replacement,* developed essentially simultaneously in Germany by Lubinus. The concept is identical to the unicompartmental replacement discussed above, except that here we are talking about the patellofemoral compartment, comprising the kneecap (patella) and the matching trochlear groove. The surgery involves less blood loss than that which is associated with a total knee replacement and the recovery is remarkably quicker. As with all forms of unicompartmental replacement, the main risk is the eventual deterioration of the other compartments, which may or may not occur in a given patient's lifetime.

> **Around the world, the popularity of partial knee replacements varies dramatically from one region to another.**

The metallic portion of today's knee replacements is made of a cobalt-chrome alloy. Titanium was used for some time but was found to be too soft to rub against the UHMWPE plastic. Experimentation is being carried out with ceramic implants and some of the metallic implants are being treated with ceramic-type surface treatments.

THE FUTURE

At some point in the future, joint replacements will be obsolete. At least for patients with arthritis. Stem cells will be injected into arthritic joints and will be activated to produce car-tilage. For now, however, surgeons and engineers are looking for implants that will last longer and provide more knee mo-tion and for tools that will allow the implantation of these re-placements through smaller incisions. Having said that, read through chapter 19 before deciding whether you want to be a joint replacement pioneer or not.

Chapter 13

❖

The Anatomy of the Knee

Anatomically the knee is more complex than the hip. For one thing, there are more moving parts.

Depending on how you count, three or four bones make up the knee (figure 13.1). There is the lower end of the *femur* (also called the thighbone), the upper end of the shinbone (*tibia*), the *kneecap* (called the patella), and the *fibula*—the little bone that runs down the side of the leg. Compared to the other bones, the fibula doesn't play a major role in knee pain or knee replacement surgery. In fact, during a knee replacement operation the surgeon never even sees the fibula.

The end of the femur features two knobs called the femoral *condyles.*

Between the knobby end of the femur and the flat, upper end of the tibia lie two cup-shaped, rubbery shock absorbers. Each one is called a *meniscus.* As discussed in the companion book in this series (*What Your Doctor May* Not *Tell You About Knee Pain and Surgery*, Warner Books, 2002), just about every MRI report will indicate that your meniscus is torn,

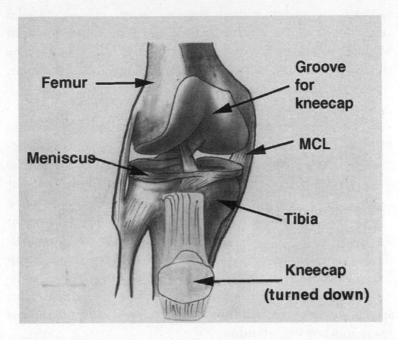

Figure 13.1 The knee joint with the patella (kneecap) turned down.

whether it is or isn't, and whether it's of any clinical significance or not.

Holding the femur and tibia together are four ligaments: the *medial collateral ligament,* the *lateral (fibular) collateral ligament,* the *anterior cruciate ligament,* and the *posterior cruciate ligament.* The knee surgeon spends half his life reconstructing the anterior cruciate ligament—as when an athlete tears it— and the other half of his life removing it—when he performs a total knee replacement!

The fleshy bulk at the front of the thigh is made up of four muscles collectively called the *quadriceps*. These muscles straighten the knee when it is bent and keep your knee from buckling when you are walking or running. At the back of the thigh one finds the hamstring muscles. These bend the knee. At the back of the knee one also finds the origin of the gastrocnemius, one of the calf muscles.

The kneecap is not attached to the lower end of the femur, but it is directly connected to the upper tibia by way of a rope-like structure called the *patellar tendon* (also called the *patellar ligament*). A tendon connects a muscle to a bone; a ligament connects two bones. Since this structure connects the kneecap to the tibia, one could legitimately call it a ligament. But since it serves to connect the quadriceps muscles to the tibia, it really functions as a tendon.

> **Not only is there cartilage under your kneecap but it's the thickest cartilage in the body.**

The ends of the femur and of the tibia are covered with articular cartilage as is the undersurface of the kneecap. In fact, measuring up to 7 millimeters, the articular cartilage of the kneecap is the thickest in the body.

When you bend and straighten your knee, the femur and tibia rotate somewhat relative to each other, as when you rotate your fist into the palm of your other hand. In other words, the knee doesn't behave like a simple hinge. This little anatomical quirk has been the bane of knee replacement surgeons and designers.

❖

Chapter 14

How Knee Replacement Surgery Is Performed

Most of you don't want to know the specifics of the operation. You've seen the operation on television and that's enough.

Some of you, however, will be curious. Here then, in broad strokes, is how it works.

You enter the operating room and a nurse called the *circulating* nurse greets you. Among many other things, he or she is in charge of getting you squared away. You'll notice someone else who is not paying attention to you. This person already has their mask and sterile gown on, and that's the *scrub nurse*. This nurse will be handing the surgeon the necessary instruments during the operation. As you enter the operating room, the scrub nurse is busy setting up.

> **The operating room is cool. This is normal, and you will quickly warm up.**

You'll note that the operating room is cool, perhaps frankly cold. That's because things warm up very quickly when the drapes are applied and the overhead operating lights are turned on. Also your surgeon will be wearing a gown and mask and it'll be a good 10 degrees warmer inside his suit. You don't want your surgeon and his team to be perspiring. If your surgeon is uncomfortable, he's more likely to want things to move along faster, which is not always to your advantage. Of equal significance is the issue of infection control. It is normal for people to shed bacteria through their clothing. Needless to say, you'd like to minimize this phenomenon near an open wound, and one way to do this is to minimize perspiration.

> **Administering antibiotics prior to surgery was once considered dangerous. Now it is routine. Specific antibiotic regimens, however, are constantly changing.**

Prior to the start of the operation, you will be given a prophylactic antibiotic by way of your intravenous (IV) line. It's called prophylactic because it is administered prior to the onset of any infection. In fact, its job is not to cure but to prevent an infection. There has been more controversy with regard to this than you might imagine. In the 1970s, it was felt that if a patient were given an antibiotic prior to surgery, he or she would simply become infected with a bacterium that was resistant to that antibiotic. Indeed no antibiotic is effective against all bacteria. The surgeons who first administered these prophylactic antibiotics took a lot of heat from their colleagues. But lo and behold, use of these antibiotics dropped the infection rate to less than 1 percent. The standard of care became to start the antibiotics before the surgery and continue them for five days thereafter ("post-op").

Surgeons cut this down to three days post-op, again taking flack from their colleagues. The current regimen consists of twenty-four hours of antibiotics with some investigators looking at just one dose before surgery. Sometimes today's malpractice is tomorrow's standard of care . . .

Choosing an antibiotic can be complex. The choice lies between an everyday broad-spectrum antibiotic that is likely to be effective against a number of common organisms versus the antibiotic most likely to be effective against the bacteria that are prevalent in that particular hospital. The infectious diseases department of the hospital will assist with that decision.

Other than your surgeon, you may notice one or two other people scurrying around. These are your surgeon's assistants, and they are setting up the tourniquet, pads, and other accoutrements of knee replacement surgery.

Anesthesia is administered in one of three ways: "general," spinal, or epidural. With general anesthesia, an intravenous medication puts you to sleep, and a plastic tube that has been gently slipped down your throat and connected to a little ventilator assures your breathing. Spinal and epidural anesthesia are closely related. A numbing medication is injected into your lower back, below the level of the spinal cord. The exact location of the tip of the needle determines whether the anesthetic is spinal or epidural. Either way, you are numb from the waist down. Intravenous medication makes you sleep during the operation, but it's not as deep a sleep as with general anesthesia, and you are breathing on your own. In the case of an epidural anesthetic, the anesthesiologist has the option of leaving a fine plastic catheter in your back through which pain medication can be administered for a day or two after the surgery. This seems like an ideal option except for the fact that the slightest displacement of the catheter makes the system ineffective. You will find a significant variation in enthusiasm for epidural anesthesia among anesthesiologists.

Needless to say, there are pros and cons to each type of anesthetic. Factors to consider include your health, the medications you are taking, your back (spine) history, the experience of the anesthesiologist in any one particular area, and, of course, your personal apprehensions. At the time of your preadmission testing (see chapter 5) you can discuss these issues with an anesthesiologist.

A catheter may or may not be placed in your bladder. The standard varies from hospital to hospital. The advantage of such a catheter is that no one (including you) has to worry about whether you'll be able to pee after the operation. The combination of being flat on your back, receiving an anesthetic, and being administered pain medication can turn this routine act into an exercise in frustration. In long cases (and cases that take longer than expected), the catheter also keeps your bladder from becoming overly distended.

The leg is now "prepped." It is scrubbed to get any dirt off and then painted with alcohol and/or an iodine solution. Drapes are applied so that the only part of your body that is visible in the operating field is the leg to be operated on. Bright lights are focused onto the planned operative site.

> **Criss-crossing incisions can pose a challenge to the joint replacement surgeon.**

After making sure that "all systems are go," the surgeon makes the incision. It is likely to go right down the middle of the knee, unless you have undergone recent surgery with a different incision. In such a case, the surgeon may be obligated to incorporate that prior incision. Criss-crossing incisions can compromise wound healing.

The surgeon must now visualize the three bones he is going to operate on: the end of the femur, the top of the tibia, and the kneecap. To that end he will remove or peel away most of the soft tissues at the upper end of the shinbone and pull the kneecap all the way to the side so as to completely pull the shinbone forward. This is called translocating the tibia. This maneuver gives the surgeon complete access to the flat upper portion of the shinbone called the *plateau* (French for "tray").

> **If the kneecap is not tracking properly, the surgeon must adjust the kneecap like a puppeteer balancing a marionette.**

Next, the surgeon will create flat surfaces of bone upon which he will fix your knee replacement. To this end he uses, ahem, a saw. A small, electrical saw, of course, but a saw nonetheless. This is where the new medical student might get a little weak in the knees.

The challenge to the surgeon is the *tensioning* of the ligaments. Remember that, contrary to the stable ball-and-socket construct of the hip joint, the knee joint is inherently unstable: take away the ligaments, and the knee consists of two round knobs rolling on a flat table. The ligaments that are left intact during knee replacement surgery must, therefore, have the proper tension. The surgeon accomplishes this through deft cuts of the bones (figure 14.1).

Having made all his cuts, "trial" implants are inserted. These look just like the real implant but they are not solidly fixed to the bone. The surgeon implants these trials to check the motion and stability of the knee. At this point he still has

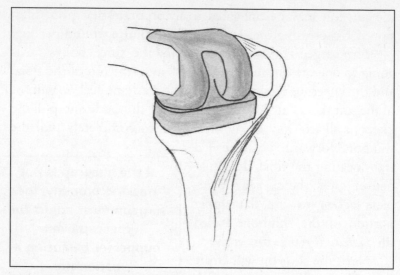

Figure 14.1 The bone is shaped to accept the implant.

the opportunity to fine-tune his cuts. The surgeon also assesses the "tracking" of the kneecap. The knee might have become arthritic as a result of kneecap malalignment, in which case the kneecap will not track down the center of the knee as the knee is flexed and straightened. If this is the case, the surgeon must adjust the kneecap like a puppeteer balancing a marionette.

Once he is satisfied, the real implants are fixed to the bone by way of cement or by way of a press-fit technique (figure 14.2).

Contrary to popular belief, orthopedic cement is not glue. It does not stick to metal or bone. Rather, it is a grout like the cement in a brick wall. It works its way into tiny interstices and locks two surfaces together.

In the press-fit technique, the implant is impacted into the

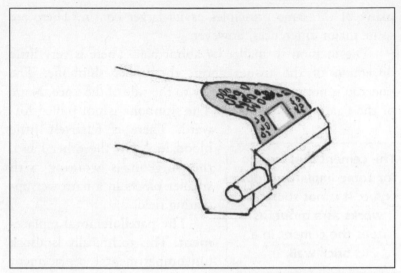

Figure 14.2. The final product. A "total knee replacement" does not take out the entire knee as the name might seem to imply. After being trimmed, the bones of the knee are covered with either metal or plastic.

bone with the expectation that bone will grow into the tiny metallic pores.

Following implantation, the incision is closed in layers as with all operations. The surgeon may or may not choose to place a drain in your knee just prior to closure. The drain keeps the knee from becoming distended with blood, but also prevents pressure from building up, pressure that in and of itself can stop the bleeding.

A dressing is applied to the knee and you are transferred to the recovery room good as new.

Partial knee replacement surgery (*unicompartmental* knee replacement). Partial knee replacement surgery follows many of the same principles as its larger cousin. There are some major differences, however.

The incision is smaller by about half. There is very little dissection of the tissues about the upper shinbone. The kneecap is not pulled completely to the side of the knee. None of the ligaments is removed. The shinbone is not pulled forward. There is relatively little blood loss. On the other hand, the surgeon is working with smaller pieces in a narrower operating field.

> **The cement that is used for some implants is not glue. It is not sticky. It works as a grout, as does the cement in a brick wall.**

The patellofemoral replacement. This technically is also a unicompartmental replacement since it replaces only one compartment, the patellofemoral compartment (kneecap). Not in the orthopedic lingo, however. The incision for a patellofemoral replacement is similar to that of a classic knee replacement. The kneecap is flipped over to expose its cartilaginous surface as is done with a total knee replacement. There is no surgical dissection around the shinbone, however, and the shinbone is not pulled forward. The femoral trochlea (groove) is sculpted to accept a metallic piece and the kneecap itself is resurfaced with the same type of plastic button used on a total knee replacement.

Chapter 15

❖

Your Hospital Stay, Day by Day

Your recovery will be smoother and less filled with anxiety if you know exactly what to expect on a day-by-day basis.

Note that the following outline may vary from surgeon to surgeon and from hospital to hospital.

If you read the previous chapter on the postoperative care of *hip* replacements, you'll naturally find a number of similarities between the protocols for the hips and the knees.

THE DAY OF SURGERY

On the day of surgery, not much is expected of you. Enjoy the rest. You'll spend a few hours in the recovery room, after which you will be transferred to your room. Regardless of the type of anesthesia, you will be groggy. The nurses will check your blood count and your vital signs, i.e., your blood pressure, temperature, pulse, and respirations. They will also check your level of pain, sometimes called the fifth vital sign.

If you have a catheter (called a Foley) in your bladder, they will monitor your urine output as a measure of how well hydrated you are, and if the surgeon has placed a drain around your knee joint, they will assess how much blood is being drained away. Your family will be allowed to visit you in the recovery room. In some recovery rooms only one person at a time is allowed in. Note that in certain hospitals the recovery room is called the PACU (Post-Anesthesia Care Unit).

POSTOPERATIVE DAY 1

Out of bed. That's the catchphrase of your first postoperative day. Be prepared not to be in the mood to do so. But it's important on many fronts: Your sense of well-being will be enhanced, your breathing will improve, your muscles will be put to use, you won't develop bedsores, you're less likely to get a rash on your back, and it will be easier to eat or drink.

> **You will be surprised to find how quickly the nurses and physical therapists get you out of bed!**

You won't walk much this first day, but the physical therapist will at least have you standing up.

You won't be very hungry, but it will be important for you to at least start taking in fluids.

If you've had a Foley catheter placed in your bladder or a drain about the knee incision, there's a good chance they'll be coming out. Although the catheter is convenient to the extent that you don't need to use a urinal or bedpan, its presence increases the risk of a urinary tract infection, which could in turn spread to your fresh knee operation.

The knee drain also presents a risk of infection. Until the

1990s, drains were considered critical. They were left in place until the amount of drainage dropped below a magic number. If the drain came out accidentally in the recovery room, that was reason enough to take the patient back to the operating room. Now it's acceptable to use a drain or not. It just goes to show how quickly the standard of care can change.

If you're not taking in much by mouth, the IV (intravenous) line will stay in your arm and provide you with fluid and basic salt.

You'll be encouraged to perform simple bed exercises. These are designed to keep the blood circulating (as opposed to pooling in your legs), to keep your muscles fresh, and to keep your lungs well expanded. Such exercises include ankle pumps, whereby you pump the ankles back and forth as if you were pushing up and down on a gas pedal, and inhaling and exhaling exercises using a small plastic incentive spirometer.

There may be a frame attached to your bed, and hanging from that frame in the neighborhood of your chest you may find a large triangle called a trapeze. This trapeze is a device that you grab when you want to lift yourself off the bed. Lifting yourself up and letting yourself back down is a good exercise.

Your pain medication will be administered by way of injections or by way of your IV. Usually you have to ask for pain medication. It's not administered automatically. The reason for this is that your doctor won't want you receiving a narcotic that you don't need. The downside to this, of course, is that nurses rarely appear the moment you call for them. My advice is to ask for pain medication as soon as you think you might need it. You are usually allowed an injection every three hours.

PCA stands for patient-controlled anesthesia. Your pain

medication is placed in a pump, and when you press a button, a small amount of pain medication flows into your vein. You press the button whenever you feel the need for pain medication. Of course, the anesthesia pain team controls how much medication is delivered with each push of the button and how many "deliveries" can take place in a given period of time.

> You will be pleased to know that pain control has (finally) become a high priority in hospitals. It is now considered the "fifth vital sign" (after pulse, respirations, heart rate, and blood pressure).

Alternate ways of administering pain medication include epidural catheters, nerve blocks (injections), and skin patches. An epidural catheter is a soft, plastic tube placed in your lower back at the time of surgery. It can be left in place after surgery, in which case an anesthetic solution is continuously allowed to drip into the epidural space. This space is near the spinal cord. A numbing medication in this area blocks the pain fibers to the legs and provides pain relief. Because the epidural space is small, the anesthesiologist may not be able to place the tip of the catheter directly into that space. Even if the catheter is perfectly placed, it may wiggle out of position after surgery when you get out of bed.

The femoral nerve high up on the thigh provides sensation to part of the knee. If that nerve is blocked by an anesthetic medication, you will obtain an element of pain relief.

Numbing medication can be pumped directly into the knee joint. This has great appeal but hasn't been fully evaluated yet.

Motion of the knee is critical after knee replacement surgery. This is one of the critical differences between a hip and a knee replacement. (Indeed, after hip replacement surgery the surgeon carefully limits the motion of the operated hip.) It takes effort to bend the knee and an equal effort to straighten it. To help you bend the knee, a CPM (*Continuous Passive Motion*) machine is placed on your bed. The machine features a cradle into which your leg is gently placed. The cradle has a hinge at the level of the knee. When the machine is turned on, the cradle automatically begins to bend and your knee bends with it. Having bent a certain distance, the cradle then straightens back out. The cycle repeats itself until you turn the machine off. Most of the time, the surgeon will want you in the CPM machine twice a day for one or two hours at a time. Every time your leg goes into the CPM, the cradle is made to bend a little more. By the time you leave the hospital, the staff would like your knee to bend as close to 90 degrees as possible (a right angle).

A freshly operated knee doesn't want to straighten out right away, but you should work hard to make sure it does. If you don't fight this trend early on, you'll find it harder and harder for the knee to cooperate. When you are not in the CPM, you should be working on this straightening, which is called *extension*.

Although it is essential for blood to clot when a wound is opened, clotting in the wrong place and at the wrong time is potentially troublesome. Patients shudder at the term *blood clot*, and although they don't exactly know why, they are correct to be concerned. Patients who undergo knee replacement surgery are at risk for developing clots in the deep veins of the leg. This condition is called (deep) phlebitis or deep vein thrombosis and is abbreviated DVT. At best you don't feel it and it is harmless. At worst, a large clot floats up through your heart and into your lung, causing a *pulmonary embolus*. This can leave you very short of breath and in extreme cases can be fatal. A number of approaches have been tried to minimize this risk. They include tablets such as warfarin and aspirin, injections of a low-molecular heparin, calf pumps, and ankle pumps, to name only the most common ones. Although all of these decrease the risk of phlebitis, it's not clear at all that they diminish the overall risk of death. Nevertheless, diminishing the risk of phlebitis is a good thing, and you'll probably find yourself receiving one of these products. Your calves, thighs, and/or feet may be wrapped in devices that inflate on a regular basis and squeeze your leg.

Blood will be drawn from your arm and sent for analysis. This will determine your blood count, i.e., it will tell the doctor the extent to which you are anemic (a certain amount of anemia is normal after a knee replacement). Your doctor may also choose to check your potassium, sodium, and other so-called chemistries.

You can expect a temperature of up to 101 degrees that may persist up to a week.

POSTOPERATIVE DAY 2

What a difference a day makes. By now you're much more with it. You'll want to know from your surgeon how the operation went and you'll want to be more active. You may even have some of your appetite back. You'll be pretty much free of tubes. And yet, you're still not yourself. You may still require shots for pain or still want the use of your PCA pump.

Today you start walking for real. The surgeon will have left instructions with respect to how much weight you can put on your operated leg, and the physical therapist will coach you in the use of a walker or crutches. How long you will need such devices depends on the specific details of your operation.

Your diet will progress to solid food if you tolerate it. If you're on a special diet, the hospital will usually be able to accommodate you. I encourage relatives to bring in a patient's favorite food. After all, poor food is how a hospital gets you out!!! Soups and shakes go down easily. No, alcohol is not allowed. But this does bring up an important point. If you're a heavy drinker, you could go into DTs (delirium tremens). It's important to let your doctors know ahead of time if you drink more than socially. And by the way, going into DTs is not a way to get your hands on a drink: you'll be treated with a sedative, not vodka.

You will still be encouraged to perform the bed exercises you were shown on Postoperative Day 1.

The timing of the first dressing change varies from hospital to hospital. It is most commonly performed on Postoperative Day

> **After this type of surgery the knee just doesn't want to move. Yet it's vital that you work on straightening the knee and bending it.**

2, 3, or 4. This dressing change will be performed by a physicians' assistant, nurse practitioner, or resident (a resident is a surgeon training to become an orthopedic surgeon). A much smaller dressing will now be applied to your incision.

Blood will again be drawn to check your level of anemia. It can take a few days for your blood count to level off. If you are on a blood thinner called Coumadin (the brand name for warfarin), a test called the INR and a test called a pro time are performed on your blood sample to check the extent to which your blood has been thinned. It can take quite a few days to find just the right dose for you. It's a tricky situation because an insufficient dose might leave you unprotected against clots while an excessive dose can lead you to bleed excessively. But the margin between one extreme and the other can be very narrow, and the medication takes two days to work. So today's blood test assesses the effect of the warfarin dose from two days ago! You can see why warfarin is not very popular. But if you are going to need a blood thinner for a few weeks or months, it's still one of the more popular options.

Using a knee immobilizer. You may find your leg wrapped in a cloth or foam device fastened with Velcro straps. Imbedded in the immobilizer are metal struts down the right and left side. These struts do not allow the immobilizer, and consequently your knee, to bend much. The immobilizer serves two purposes: First, it keeps your knee relatively straight. This is important because the operated knee wants to remain somewhat bent, and if it remains bent twenty-four hours a day, you'll be disappointed to find that it becomes increasingly difficult to straighten.

Second, a knee that's been operated on is painful and can feel unsteady during simple walking. The immobilizer provides security by not allowing the knee to buckle. Of course, the immobilizer must be removed before the leg is placed back in the CPM machine!

Here is an oft-overlooked point: In order to be effective, the immobilizer must be applied correctly. I invite you to make rounds with me (not really) and we'll count the number of patients whose immobilizer is properly positioned. The middle of the immobilizer must be at the level of the knee. If it is wrapped around your calf with the top of the immobilizer resting about the knee, it is useless. And yet because an immobilizer can indeed slide down the leg if it's not tight enough, that's where the surgeon often finds the darn device as he makes rounds on the orthopedic wing of the hospital. It's an even bigger problem in nursing homes, where the staff is less attuned to these subtleties and patients may not have as much wherewithal.

POSTOPERATIVE DAY 3

You are now free of tubes. Under supervision you will start to get out of bed by yourself.

You will start to walk up and down the hallway. There may be some pain, but it will be very different from your preoperative pain: you will note surgical soreness, as opposed to the grinding, lancing pain you experienced before.

At this point your pain medication will consist of pills, freeing you up from IVs and injections.

The anticoagulation measures will still be in effect, as they will be during your whole hospital stay.

Depending on the hospital setting, you might be able to shower.

Expect swelling in the operated leg. It does not mean that you have developed blood clots. In fact, the correlation between blood clots and leg swelling is poor. For this reason your surgeon may choose to automatically obtain a *duplex* test that examines your leg for clots. These duplex tests are kinder, gentler versions of a *venogram,* whereby dye is injected into a vein. A duplex test is painless.

Your team will be checking the amount of drainage present on your dressing. It should taper off on a daily basis.

If you are cleared by physical therapy and if the drainage from your wound has essentially ceased, you might be discharged from the hospital later in the day or tomorrow morning.

POSTOPERATIVE DAY 4

If you were still somewhat groggy or unsteady on Day 3, or if your wound still exhibited significant drainage, your surgeon will keep you in the hospital. The presence of drainage may or may not lead your surgeon to put you back on antibiotics. This is a controversial area.

The routine will be the same: getting out of bed, walking, learning to become more independent, anticoagulation, etc.

POSTOPERATIVE DAY 5

This is another potential day of discharge. You will need clearance from the physical therapist and your wound will need to be essentially dry.

Persistent drainage can eventually lead to an infection, and your surgeon may choose to take you back to the operating room to wash out whatever it is that is draining *before* it becomes infected.

AFTER THE HOSPITAL

When you leave the hospital, you will either go home or be transferred to an inpatient rehabilitation facility. This rehabilitation unit might be in a hospital (such as the one you are already in) or in a nursing home (skilled nursing facility).

Either way, you want to be clear on the plans, precautions, and danger signs. The plans will include follow-up with your doctor, therapy you are supposed to receive, and medications you are supposed to take. Precautions include telling the doctors and dentists taking care of you to note in their chart that you have a knee replacement. Danger signs include a temperature of 101 degrees or greater, increasing redness about the incision, increasing swelling (remember: some swelling is normal), increasing pain, and any kind of drainage. Some health professionals are not aware of the risks posed by persistent oozing. They are falsely reassured by the fact that the drainage consists of clear liquid and doesn't appear to be infected.

You should go home with some basic equipment—or at least obtain it very soon upon arriving home. This includes a grabber to help you pick objects off the floor and a raised toilet seat. Devices also exist to assist you with putting on socks.

Chapter 16

❖

Going Home After Knee Replacement Surgery

Gee, it's good to be back home. The hospital wasn't so bad after all, but it's nice to be home. If nothing else, it's good to be in your own bed and not be disturbed by all those hospital noises. Heck, get up when you feel like it.

Now is the time to put into practice everything you learned in the hospital.

EXERCISING AFTER KNEE REPLACEMENT SURGERY

Although your surgeon was deft and delicate as he fashioned your knee to accept the implant, your knee still feels that it's been attacked. It remains somewhat stiff and swollen, and the benefits of the operation may not be obvious yet. First and foremost, you still need to exercise.

Exercises are divided into three categories: range-of-motion exercises, strengthening, and functional training.

Range of Motion

Range of motion is the term used by surgeons and therapists to denote the extent of bending and straightening you are capable of. Straightening is called *extension* and bending is called *flexion.* Your therapist will try to bring you to "full extension," meaning that he or she will want your knee to fully straighten. At the other extreme, your therapist will try to get you to bend the knee as much as possible. These range-of-motion exercises are critical. Indeed, as the weeks go by, it becomes harder to achieve greater motion as a result of the normal scarring of tissues that takes place. *Scar* is dense tissue with very little give to it, and it's a normal component of healing. Some people form more scar tissue than others. The goal is to achieve all the motion you are going to get before this scar tissue gels or sets, so to speak.

> **Exercising is divided into range of motion, strengthening, and functional training.**

Although the therapist will work with you, most of the work is carried out by *you* throughout the day.

To straighten the knee, you can either perform quadriceps setting exercises ("quad sets") or use the following trick: Lie on your stomach with the knee right at the edge of the bed. The weight of your leg will gradually stretch your knee until it is straight. If your leg is too light, you can wrap an ankle weight around it, or a pocketbook filled with books (ten copies of this book make a perfect weight).

Here's how you perform a quad set: Lie on your back, and tighten your leg muscles until the back of your leg touches the bed or whatever else you are lying on. Count to 10. Relax. Start again.

Strengthening

The term *strengthening* is self-explanatory. As you use your muscles, they become stronger. The key to any strengthening program is, therefore, to work your muscles a little harder than what they've been used to, and this usually means lifting or pushing a weight. Then there is isometric exercise: You tighten muscles without moving. The *quad set is an example of such an isometric exercise.*

Quad sets offer three benefits to patients who have undergone knee replacement surgery: They provide an element of strengthening, they help you reach full extension if you haven't done so yet, and they help pump the blood in your legs back to your heart. This pumping action keeps the venous blood from stagnating and minimizes the risk of blood clots forming deep within the leg. Ankle pumps, an exercise whereby you pump your foot up and down as if it were on the gas pedal of a car, are even better at pumping blood back to your heart. Ankle pumps, however, do not provide much strengthening.

Your leg makes for a pretty good weight, and so a basic knee exercise is to lie on your back and raise your leg, count to 10, and let it down. This is called straight leg raising. The first time around, you won't be able to hold the leg up for 10 seconds. Do what you can and progressively work up to 10 seconds. *Caution:* (1) This can stress your back. If you are prone to back pain or sciatica (a pinched nerve down the leg), back off on this exercise at the first hint of pain. (2) This exercise places high stresses on the patellar tendon, the flat, ribbon-like tendon connecting your kneecap to your tibia. In rare cases this tendon can rupture. I've never seen this happen, but it has been reported. Patients who take prednisone or other steroids have weaker tendons and are at risk for this complication as are patients who have just undergone a repeat knee reconstruction (the tendons become less resilient with each operation). A particularly heavy leg might also predispose to a tendon rupture. In these special cases I recommend holding off on straight leg raising exercises for six weeks.

Functional Training

Functional training means that you simulate activities that are important to you. Walking, for example. The best way to simulate walking is, well, to walk. Not only do you strengthen your muscles, but you retrain your muscles to work in concert. The analogy to music is appropriate: All members of an orchestra must work with seamless precision to produce a harmonious sound, and all muscles about the leg must work with equal harmony to produce a smooth gait.

> **Walking in the shallow end of a swimming pool is an outstanding exercise.**

If you have access to a swimming pool, walking in the shallow end is an outstanding exercise. Because you are buoyant, you place little stress on the operated knee, and the resistance of the water provides a reasonable challenge to the knee and thigh muscles. For variety, try walking backward and sideways. You may also use a kickboard or swim. Both the freestyle and the breast stroke are acceptable.

DRIVING, SEX, ETC.

In order to drive, you must be able to comfortably go from the gas to the brake pedal, and that is the limiting factor in your return to driving.

If your left knee was operated on and you drive with your right foot, you can drive anytime—assuming your mental faculties are not diminished by pain or by pain medication.

Sexual activity is limited only by pain and imagination.

HOME PRECAUTIONS

Hopefully you'll have gotten your home ready *prior* to the surgery, but it's not too late to do so now.

A bath mat and wall handles are a good idea since a shower tends to be a slippery place.

Your foot can get caught in throw rugs, and your balance isn't back to normal, so have the rugs removed.

Don't walk in the dark. Turn on a light if you must get up at night, and you'll avoid tripping on that shoe.

BILATERAL KNEE REPLACEMENT (BOTH KNEES)

If you've had both knees replaced during the same hospitalization, the protocols remain the same. Obviously you need to expend even more time on exercising although some exercises can be performed simultaneously. Both knees can be placed in a CPM machine, you can lie on your stomach to extend both knees simultaneously, and you can perform quad sets on both sides at the same time.

At first, all of your energy will be directed to your operated knee(s). As time passes, your attention will gradually return to your everyday activities and the knees will gradually become a secondary issue. The time it takes you to forget that you've undergone surgery is highly variable. A minimum would be three months and for some people it can take as long as a year. When all is said and done, chances are you'll be happy you underwent the procedure.

Part IV

———

CONTROVERSIES
AND
ADMONITIONS

Chapter 17

❧

Do's and Don'ts After Surgery

A joint replacement, whether it be a hip or a knee replacement, is a sturdy device designed to be treated like a delicate object. You hope it will last a lifetime, keeping in mind that all mechanical devices can eventually wear out.

RULE 1. DON'T run or jump any more than you have to.

The weak link is the bearing, in other words the parts that are rubbing together. The more the parts rub, the quicker they wear out. Also, if the joint replacement has been cemented into the bone, the cement can weaken and crack over time. The more stress that is placed on the implant, the faster the cement will crack.

RULE 2. If you are undergoing dental or bowel procedures, DO tell the doctor or dentist that you have a joint replacement.

Bacteria from distant parts of the body can settle into a joint. These bacteria stick to the metal or plastic part of the implant, and the body can't fight them off. The dirtiest parts of the body are the bowel and the mouth. Therefore, your doctor or dentist will prescribe an antibiotic to be taken before and/or after the procedure. This is called a *prophylactic* antibiotic. Exception: The current thinking is that a routine dental cleaning more than a year after surgery carried out in a person without medical problems (diabetes, for example) does *not* require prophylactic antibiotics.

RULE 3. DON'T worry about undergoing an MRI (magnetic resonance imaging) test, unless your doctor tells you that you have other contraindications for one. The metal used in joint replacements is nonmagnetic and consequently there will be no magnetic tug on the implant.

Having said this, keep in mind that the metal of your implant causes "scatter" that makes it difficult if not impossible to read an MRI study performed in the vicinity of the replacement.

If your hip hurts after a joint replacement, an MRI of the hip is unlikely to be helpful. An MRI of your back, though, might be perfectly reasonable (since hip pain can come from the back), and such an MRI would be perfectly readable even in the presence of a hip replacement.

RULE 4. Following hip replacement surgery, when sitting, DON'T bend forward or twist your upper body without thinking of your hip replacement. One of the most sudden and painful complications of a hip replacement is a dislocation, where the ball of the hip replacement suddenly pops out.

The hip should not be bent more than 90 degrees (a right

angle). Consequently, if you are sitting in a chair, DON'T bend forward to get up. Scoot to the edge and then get up.

If you are in a car and something falls under the seat, DON'T reach underneath to find it.

If the phone rings, DON'T reach way forward and across your body to answer it.

DO sit in the highest possible chairs. DON'T settle into a chaise longue or a deep recliner without thinking of how you are going to get out.

When you sit, the operated leg must be abducted. That means that it must point away from the midline. The right leg points to the right, the left leg to the left. The knee can be straight or bent. *The lower you sit and the more you lean forward, the more important this becomes.*

In short, though you shouldn't lean forward when you sit, you can usually get away with it if the operated leg is abducted.

If you are standing, do not drop your head below your waist.

If you are standing and need to pick something off the floor, DO use a grabber, and/or DO move the operated leg behind you or off to the side.

These are lifetime precautions. Some patients do not dislocate their hip until many years after their operation, when they aren't so vigilant about protecting their joint replacement.

Since these concepts can be a little tricky, do not hesitate to question your physical therapist and surgeon until you've got it right. In time, these precautions will become second nature.

RULE 5. DO remember to take your blood thinner (a pill or an injection). Blood coming back to the heart courses through veins, those blue structures you see on the back of your hands. (The veins that you can see are called *superficial* veins; those that lie deep inside your legs, arms, and pelvis are termed *deep*). As noted in chapter 18, clots can form in these veins and these clots are associated with medical complications varying from leg swelling to sudden and eternal sleep.

Anticoagulation may or may not be as necessary for partial knee replacements carried out through incisions that are smaller than those of a complete replacement.

The exact nature of the blood thinner and how long you need to take it are subjects of great controversy. If you are at risk for stomach ulcers or any kind of bleeding from the bowel, the risks of taking a blood thinner may outweigh the benefits. This is a tricky issue that your surgeon and family doctor will have to wrestle with.

RULE 6. DO keep your follow-up appointments. As time goes by, it is easy to forget certain precautions (Rule 4, for instance). The follow-up appointment is an opportunity for a refresher course.

If your hip and knee feel well, chances are that your replacement is functioning as it should. But as noted in greater detail in chapter 18, silent problems can exist. Osteolysis can be taking place, a process by which the bone around your implant withers away. Also the bearing surfaces (the surfaces that rub together) can eventually wear down. Since, in time, these processes become visible on a plain X-ray, it makes sense to see your surgeon on a regular basis.

Unlike dentists, orthopedists do not routinely send yearly reminders to their patients, though it wouldn't be a bad idea. Alternatively, make the appointment a year ahead of time as you are leaving your surgeon's office. A few days before that next appointment, the call from your doctor confirming your appointment will serve as your yearly reminder. You can always reschedule.

RULE 7. DO make your house as safe as possible: Falling and breaking a bone is never fun. But breaking a bone near a joint replacement is much worse. It often results in difficult surgery. To the extent that you can, the key is to avoid the break in the first place. Fractures (the medical term for a break) occur most commonly around the house. This is not surprising since this is where we spend most of our time. So remove items that you are likely to trip over. That includes throw rugs, extension cords, and the like. Install grab bars in the bath/shower area as well as bath mats.

RULE 8. At the risk of disturbing your mate, DO NOT get up at night without turning on the light.

RULE 9. DO get your eyes checked on a regular basis. Improper lens prescriptions for eyeglasses can lead to falls.

RULE 10. DO think positive. Your hip and knee aren't good as new. You're not twenty years old again. But much of the pain you had before surgery should be gone, and you must focus on what's improved rather than on what could still be better.

Chapter 18

Complications

This is perhaps the most difficult chapter for me to write and the most demanding subject for your surgeon to discuss. He hates to discourage you from an operation that has a very good chance of turning your life around for the better, but at the same time you need to be an informed consumer. If your surgeon doesn't spend enough time discussing complications, then he hasn't done his job with respect to educating you. On the other hand, if he dwells too long on the subject, you are going to think that he is Doctor Doom and Gloom and that he is not the doctor for you.

Wherefore the advantage of this book. I can spend all the time I want discussing complications, and you are free to pore over every word or skip to another chapter.

INFECTION

I'll start right off with the most feared complication. It is difficult to impart upon a patient the seriousness of an infection in the setting of a joint replacement. We tend to think of infections as conditions that are treated with ten days of antibiotics, but it's not so easy with a joint replacement.

How do you know if you have an infection? Sometimes it's easy: You have a fever and pus is oozing from the wound. But most of the time, it's not so obvious. Perhaps there's just some harmless-looking clear liquid coming from the incision.

> It is difficult to overstate the seriousness of an infection in the setting of a joint replacement.

In fact, if you notice such a liquid more than ten days or so after your surgery, you should alert your surgeon, for persistent drainage can lead to an infection. Your main symptom may simply be pain. But any number of conditions can cause pain around your hip or knee, most of which are much more common (and less serious) than an infection. Since some pain is normal for three months or so after surgery, your surgeon will wait until you've reached that milestone before looking into the possibility of an infection.

> Clear liquid coming from an incision is not a good sign in someone who has undergone a joint replacement.

What he won't do is simply prescribe antibiotics.

There are a number of reasons for this: First, in order to work, antibiotics have to reach the offending bacteria. They do so by way of the bloodstream. But the surgical site is often encased in scar tissue, tissue that features very few blood vessels. Therefore, the antibiotics may not reach the infected area. Second, some bacteria literally stick to the implant. It's as if they had arms to wrap around the darn thing. The antibiotics just can't penetrate the sticky coating around the bacteria. Third, different bacteria respond to different antibiotics. If your doctor doesn't know what type of bacteria is involved, he doesn't know specifically which antibiotics to order. Finally, antibiotics will make it difficult for a laboratory to grow (culture) and identify the bacteria.

Believe it or not, there is no single foolproof test to definitively tell the doctor whether you are brewing an infection.

> **There is no single test that always rules an infection in or out.**

Tests that your doctor will consider include blood tests (CBC, sed rate [ESR], CRP), nuclear scans (technetium, gallium, indium), and aspirations. Nuclear scans involve the injection of a slightly radioactive product into your arm. You return to the nuclear medicine doctor anywhere from three hours to two days later and are placed in a Geiger counter type of device. It's not a tunnel, so you don't have to worry about claustrophobia. It's painless. The test looks for "hot spots." The pattern of the hot spots suggests to the doctor the presence or absence of an infection. The reliability of these nuclear tests is subject to debate.

For an aspiration, the doctor takes fluid from the joint and sends it for analysis. This analysis includes a culture. The laboratory looks for bacteria and tries to get them to grow so they can be identified. Usually a negative culture means that there are no bacteria; therefore, you don't have an infection. A positive culture implies that there are bacteria in your joint and that you are harboring an infection. However, there exist so-called false positives and negatives. An infection can exist in the absence of a positive culture, as when a patient is already on antibiotics, and a positive culture can exist even though there is no infection. This happens when bacteria from the skin or from the air contaminate the culture. All these tests are pieces of a puzzle. The doctor pieces these tests together until a picture emerges. If every test strongly suggests the presence or absence of an infection, the surgeon will be able to give you a relatively definite diagnosis. But if the tests are equivocal or point in different directions, the surgeon (and you) have some difficult decisions to make.

Surgeons divide infections into different categories: an infection is called *acute* if it occurs soon after your surgery. It is termed *chronic* if it occurs sometime after the operation. I am deliberately vague here, because there is some disagreement as to where to draw the line between acute and chronic. Moreover, if the time of the infection can be specifically determined (e.g., two days after the extraction of an infected tooth), and the joint infection is detected very quickly, this might also qualify as an acute infection, even though the operation took place a long time ago. The distinction between an acute and a chronic infection is critical, for the treatment will be quite different.

Either way, an infected implant is your ticket to ride back to the operating theater. In the case of an acute infection, the bacteria have not had the opportunity to burrow into the bone, and the surgical site "simply" needs to be cleaned. If it is a knee that is infected, the surgeon might choose to wash out the joint by way of an arthroscopy. This operation requires no more than a few tiny incisions, through which the surgeon inserts fine tubes and instruments. Quarts of fluid are run through the knee, and inflamed, angry-looking tissue can be shaved away.

The orthopedic community has not come to an agreement on exactly which patients are candidates for this arthroscopic washout, but, by and large, the more acute the infection (the sooner it is detected from the time it begins), the older and more frail the patient, and the milder the bacteria, the greater the odds that the surgeon will recommend an arthroscopic approach. Alternatively, your incision will be opened (pretty much the whole length of it), and the surgeon will work his way down into the joint much the same way he did the first time around. The surgeon will wash out the area with a saline solution using a Water Pik type of jet lavage to dislodge those stubborn bacteria. He may choose to remove parts of the implant that can be exchanged without requiring hours of destructive surgery, and he then replaces these parts with fresh ones.

> **An infection usually leads to at least one other operation.**

Following the operation, your surgeon will place you on three to twelve weeks of antibiotics. These antibiotics will consist of either pills or of intravenous injections, and your blood will be drawn and monitored on a regular basis.

And that's the good news.

If you are deemed to have a chronic infection, things are even worse (last chance to get off here and go to another chapter).

In the case of a chronic infection, the entire implant will probably have to come out. Because of the enormity of this procedure, your surgeon might first try the washout approach described above. Following this he might place you on antibiotics for months, perhaps even forever. This doesn't cure the infection; it "suppresses" it. The bacteria are still there, but they lie dormant. Removing the implant isn't easy. Imagine removing a brick from a wall without disturbing the surrounding bricks. The surgeon must remove the implant without damaging the surrounding bone. Once this has been done, the surgeon is faced with two choices: he can clean the surgical site and implant a new replacement (this is called a *primary exchange*), or clean the site, place you on antibiotics for a few weeks, and come back another day to implant a new prosthesis. It's a toss-up between pleasing you in the short run and leaving you satisfied in the long run. Indeed, the first option allows you to leave the hospital with a functioning implant, but if sufficient bacteria remain, the infection could develop all over again. The second option is more painful psychologically in that you leave the hospital without a functioning implant. You are walking around with crutches, and the doctor won't allow you to put much weight on the leg. This complicates most aspects of daily living. This second option, on the other hand, improves the odds of curing the surgical site of its infection before a joint replacement is reimplanted. To determine whether to choose the first or second option, the surgeon will consider many factors, including your health, your age, and your obligations in life. Most important of all, however, is the exact nature of the bacteria involved. Some are more tenacious and difficult to treat, and the presence of such bacteria will make your surgeon lean toward Option 2. On the other hand, the presence of less virulent bacteria may induce your surgeon to go for the "primary exchange" option.

> **If the implant has to be removed, a new implant can sometimes be inserted during the same operation.**

What can you do to prevent an infection? Alert the doctor to the presence of drainage (liquid coming from the wound) even if the liquid appears to be no more than water. Eat well. I didn't say eat a lot. I said eat *well.* You want a healthy mix of foods. If your appetite isn't great, consider milk shake–like products that your doctor or pharmacist can point you to in order to take in an adequate amount of calories, vitamins, and minerals.

BLOOD CLOTS

Deep venous thrombosis/phlebitis/blood clots/pulmonary embolus—these scary words are all variations on a theme.

Deep inside a person's leg lie veins that carry blood back to the heart and to the lungs. Sometimes a clot will form on the inner wall of one of these veins. This is called *deep venous thrombosis,* commonly abbreviated *DVT.*

Like streams feeding a river, small veins in the legs merge with larger veins until they all spill into the vena cava, the large pipe that returns blood to the heart. This blood is dark red, having given up its oxygen. The heart now pumps this blood into the lungs by way of the pulmonary artery. The pulmonary artery splits into two, sending half the blood to each lung. Now replenished with oxygen, the bright red blood returns to the heart, where it is pumped out via the aorta to the rest of the body.

> **Patients undergoing hip or knee replacement surgery are at particular risk for developing DVT.**

Patients undergoing hip and knee replacement surgery are at particular risk for DVT for reasons that are only partly understood. In fact, generally speaking, the condition is incompletely understood. Particularly frustrating is its apparent randomness. Even young, seemingly healthy patients who are not undergoing major hip or knee surgery can develop the condition.

Very often DVT is asymptomatic, in other words, it causes no symptoms. The patient is completely unaware that the condition exists. Sometimes the offending clot will cause the leg to swell and to be painful, in which case a person is said to suffer from *phlebitis*. Keep in mind that there exists a similar condition called *superficial phlebitis* involving the superficial veins of the leg, the veins that you see right there under your skin. Superficial phlebitis is *not* associated with serious blood clots.

In a small percentage of patients with DVT, the clot will break off and make its way to the lungs. Remember that the lungs replenish oxygen-depleted blood. The clot acts as a plug and blocks the circulation to a part of the lungs. This is called a *pulmonary embolus.* That leaves less lung to reoxygenate blood. The patient may still not feel a thing if the embolus is small and only a small portion of the lung has been knocked out. Some patients, though, will experience shortness of breath, sweating, or chest pain. This is a medical emergency. More emboli might follow, a situation that can eventually be fatal. The treatment for a pulmonary embolus consists of breathing oxygen and taking a blood thinner that will dissolve existing clots and prevent the creation of new ones. If a clot is large enough, it can block out both lungs, a situation that causes a person to quickly pass out and pass away.

The prevention of blood clots. Every surgeon who performs hip and knee replacement surgery is acutely aware of the DVT risks. You will, therefore, be placed on some form of prophylaxis, a regimen designed to minimize the risks. What you really need to appreciate is that this is a very controversial area that your surgeon will not have time to fully go over with you. There is controversy over what treatment to provide and for how long. Treatment options include medications and leg pumps. The medications include little injections given right under the skin (Lovenox, Fragmin, and Arixtra to name but a few) and pills, such as warfarin (Coumadin) and aspirin. The pumps include thigh pumps, calf pumps, and foot pumps. The medications can be combined with pumps. Now you begin to see how many possible combinations exist. Add to this the fact that the regimen you are on in the hospital might not be practical at home. And nobody knows for sure how long you need to be on this type of prophylaxis. The party line is, up to twelve weeks.

> There is no ideal way to prevent blood clots.

What muddies the waters is that every treatment is associated with its own set of complications. If you thin someone's blood to prevent clotting, a serious bleed can ensue. That bleed might take place soon after surgery in the freshly operated knee or hip. Or it might present itself in the form of a bleeding ulcer.

In any given patient, the surgeon must weigh the risk of one complication over another.

As you might imagine, doctors can be rather opinionated on this matter. One doctor will swear by an injectable blood thinner, a second one will routinely use aspirin, another will prescribe foot pumps, and yet another may combine these options or start with one and then switch to another.

One small item that is poorly appreciated even by the

medical community is that with regard to preventing *death,* none of the pharmacological agents is truly effective. They simply swap one cause of death for another. Without a blood thinner on board, a patient has a very small chance of *dying* from a blood clot. With a blood thinner, they stand a very small chance of dying from a complication of the medication. And the risks are about the same. This is not just my opinion. This conclusion was published as the lead article and editorial in a very respected orthopedic journal.

Pharmacological agents are, however, effective in diminishing the risks of phlebitis and nonfatal pulmonary emboli.

The cost and complications of pharmacological agents have spurred interest in leg and foot pumps. Throughout the day and night the leg pumps inflate and deflate every few seconds while the foot pumps impart an impact on the sole of the foot. These keep the venous blood from stagnating and clotting. There is a sound associated with the use of these devices, and while some might find it soothing and hypnotic, to others it is a form of Chinese water torture. Also some find the foot pumps to be outright uncomfortable. The search for the perfect anticoagulation regimen continues.

> **Preventing heart disease and preventing DVT require different doses of aspirin.**

There is a misconception pertaining to aspirin that I would like to go over with you. Aspirin for the prevention of heart disease is often prescribed as "baby aspirin" once a day, i.e., one 81-milligram tablet a day. For the prevention of clots in the large veins of the legs and pelvis, a full adult pill (325 milligrams) twice a day is the recommended dose. It is perfectly acceptable to take the aspirin in a coated form.

Filters. No, not cigarette filters. A filter is a device placed in the vena cava, the large vessel that brings blood back to the heart. The filter literally catches the clots before they can make their way to the heart and to the lungs. A filter is placed in someone at particularly high risk for DVT and/or a patient who cannot tolerate a blood thinner. You won't be surprised to discover that these filters also have their complications. They can cause leg swelling, and a clot can occasionally slip around the filter. In summary, everybody recognizes the risks of DVT in patients undergoing hip and knee replacement surgery, but no one has come up with a risk-free way of avoiding it. If you have a particular aversion to the regimen recommended by your doctor, at least know that other options exist.

WOUND DRAINAGE

Abe had surgery two weeks ago. A bit of clear liquid is coming from the surgical site. Perhaps it's coming from the little pinhole where a drain used to be; perhaps it's in the middle of a persistent scab. Either way, as innocuous as it looks, it's a *major problem*. Either there's an infection brewing or an infection is bound to develop. Sooner or later a communication between the outside world and a joint replacement will lead to an infection. Once you have left the hospital, your job is to let your doctor know that this is taking place. He will want it evaluated ASAP, and don't be surprised if he tells you that he's taking you to the operating room to wash out the joint with a Water Pik type of irrigation device. If it looks as if you already have an infection, your surgeon may well remove and replace ("exchange") the plastic part of the implant, i.e., the portion of the implant that can often be exchanged without ruining the whole construct (see

"Infection," above). Even this can be challenging at times, and the surgeon has to weigh the pros and cons of this approach.

STIFFNESS

A knee that is traumatized does not want to move, and yes, the knee considers replacement surgery to be trauma, though inflicted with the best of intentions. The knee is happy to remain slightly bent and it will resist attempts to have it straightened or bent any further. Therefore, both patient and therapist must perform considerable work to get the knee going. In some patients, the knee simply refuses to bend as much as it should, even after much physical therapy. In this case, the surgeon may elect to perform a *manipulation* in the operating room if the motion is truly unsatisfactory. During a manipulation, the surgeon gently bends the knee to the desired position. Because the procedure is performed under anesthesia, it is painless. There are risks, of course. If the surgeon pushes just a little too hard or if the tissues are weaker than normal, something might break. The surgeon might want to combine the manipulation with an *arthroscopy*. For this operation, the surgeon places two or three small holes about the knee through which he inserts pencil-like instruments. These instruments allow him to see inside the knee and to remove the scar tissue that is blocking your motion (see *What Your Doctor May* Not *Tell You About Knee Pain and Surgery*, Warner Books, 2002).

> Getting the knee to bend after knee surgery is a team effort among patient, physical therapist, and surgeon. Sometimes even that isn't enough.

PERSISTENT SCABS

It's not uncommon to have small scabs over part of the incision. These are thin, narrow scabs directly over the incision and are not worrisome. Particularly in knees, however, a round scab can indicate that the incision has not healed. Directly under that scab lies not skin but your kneecap or its tendon. That poses a potential problem.

> Do not pick at scabs along the incision.

The day that scab comes off, the outside world is communicating with your knee, and once again, you are at risk for developing an infection. *So do not pick scabs!* Make sure your surgeon is aware of their presence. You may require a skin or a muscle graft to cover that part of the incision (a big operation!). It's always easier to take care of conditions before they become emergencies. Did I say this already? DO NOT PICK SCABS!

HETEROTOPIC OSSIFICATION

This is becoming as rare as it is difficult to pronounce. It is abbreviated HO. It's much more a complication of hip surgery than knee surgery, but even in hips it's now unusual. I say "now" because once upon a time it bordered on being common, and quite a few articles have been written about this. Why we've see this welcome trend nobody knows for sure.

In patients with HO, bone forms in places where it doesn't belong. It's incredible to think that we cannot readily strengthen osteoporotic bones (bones lacking in bony substance), yet there goes bone forming in places it has no business being! If we knew exactly how to turn on this bone-forming signal, we'd cure osteoporosis.

HO around the hip involves the abductor muscles, pretty much where the top of your pants pocket might be. HO ranges from mild to severe (Grade I to Grade IV, in medical lingo). In its mildest forms, parts of the muscle turn to bone, but not enough for you to ever notice. It's strictly an x-ray finding, and a medical curiosity. But in its severest form (Grade IV), the entire abductor muscle has turned to bone, and now it limits your hip's mobility. It can also be painful. Fortunately Grade IV HO is rare.

Prevention is key, but as with DVT (see above) there is no easy, inexpensive, risk-free prevention. Anti-inflammatory medications (NSAIDs) can work, as can radiation. NSAIDs can cause ulcers, though, especially if you are taking a blood thinner, and radiation can conceivably slow the bone ingrowth that you are *trying* to achieve around your implant. It's also emotionally unappealing to receive a dose of radiation anywhere if you don't really need it!

The surgeon will evaluate the need for HO prevention on a case-by-case basis. Big, young men are statistically more at risk, but again it is a condition we see far less frequently than in the early days of joint replacement surgery. One of the theories is that in the last twenty years surgeons have used Water Pik type of devices to intermittently clean the operative site, something that did not exist in the earlier years. These water jets remove the tiny bits of near-invisible bone gradually distributed throughout the hip or knee during the operation. It is conceivable that these tiny bony bits stimulate the formation of HO, and by removing them, the risk of HO greatly diminishes.

Here's an interesting medical tidbit for you to chew on if you are scientifically inclined: Patients with head trauma are at risk for developing severe HO around the hip in the absence of any hip surgery or injury! Go figure!

PERSISTENT PAIN

D.S. is fifty-five years old. He's been crippled with arthritis for many years and has finally given in to hip replacement surgery. One year later he's far better than he was before surgery. He can work as an oral surgeon and can walk to and from the center of town. His thigh aches, however, when he gets up from a sitting position. He doesn't feel he can run or play tennis.

I.N. is seventy-six years old. It's been eight months since her knee replacement. Her friends all tell her that she should be better by now, but she isn't. She's starting to wonder if the problem is with her. Is she overly demanding? Is she overly sensitive? But sometimes she gets angry. Did the surgeon do something wrong? Was he really the one who performed the surgery? Was he there the whole time? Was the insurance reimbursement too low for him?

The above scenarios are taken from real patients, patients who typically seek many opinions once they're convinced that something isn't right. It's difficult to say what percentage of patients fall into this category. We know roughly what percentage of implants are revised (redone), but that doesn't account for the patients who simply live with a degree of pain. My educated guess is that 5 percent of patients fall into this category. Surgeons are not the best judges of this, for their problem patients may go elsewhere for treatment, leaving them with only their best results.

Faced with a patient complaining of pain, the surgeon treads a fine line between being reassuring and being dismissive. This is especially true in the first few months after surgery. Indeed, the tissues can remain sore for quite some time and this masks the pain-relieving aspects of the surgery.

After approximately three months, the bulk of the pain should have resolved. If significant pain persists beyond that time, the surgeon must now start to consider a work-up, in other words, an investigation. As with any investigation, the surgeon looks for the suspects. These include: an infection, loosening of the implant, allergy to one of the metallic components, pain coming from a different part of the body, and neurological conditions such as neuromas, reflex sympathetic dystrophy, and neuropathies.

> **Faced with a patient complaining of pain, the surgeon treads a fine line between being reassuring and being dismissive.**

An infection is worrisome for the reasons outlined at the beginning of the chapter, and it need not present itself with classic signs of infection such as redness and fever. It can be very difficult and in some cases outright impossible to diagnose an infection without actually taking out the implant, and that is no small matter.

A cemented implant is unlikely to have loosened so early on, but a cementless implant may not have "taken." In other words, bone has not grown into the small interstices of the rough surface and has not captured the implant. With every step, the implant moves ever so slightly and causes pain. This may or may not be visible on the X-ray. Among other things, the surgeon will look for signs that the implant has changed position.

Pain in the hip can radiate down from the pelvis or back, as can pain in the knee. Knee pain can come from the hip. This is called *referred pain,* a phenomenon where abnormalities in one part of the body cause pain at a more distant site. It happens everywhere in the body: A pinched nerve in the neck can cause shoulder pain, a rotator cuff tear in the shoulder leads to upper-arm pain, etc. You don't want to undergo multiple hip operations only to find that the pain was coming from a herniated disk in your back.

> **Pain in the knee can be caused by a hip, back, or nerve problem!**

Pain is transmitted from your leg to your brain by way of nerves. Anything that irritates those nerves is read by your brain as "knee pain" or "hip pain" even if there is nothing wrong with your knee or hip. This is an important point that calls for elaboration. Imagine that there were just one nerve, just one pain fiber, going from your brain to your right big toe. If you were to stub your big toe, a message would race up to your brain via that one pain fiber and your brain would register "pain in big right toe."

> **RSD is a strange condition associated with unrelenting pain.**

Now here's the catch: If you were to pinch that pain fiber at any point between your big toe and brain, say in the middle of your back, your brain would again register "pain in big right toe"! There's nothing wrong with your big toe!

Let's get back to the painful hip or knee replacement. Irritation of a nerve going from your knee or hip to your brain will cause you to feel pain in your knee or hip. The back is the most common source of referred pain to the hip or knee.

REFLEX SYMPATHETIC DYSTROPHY

This mouthful of a condition goes by a number of names and abbreviations, including RSD, complex regional pain syndrome, CRPS, algodystrophy, and causalgia. It is a somewhat mysterious condition where the pain fibers are continuously stimulated. It's the equivalent of persistent sneezing even after the pepper's been removed from under your nose. The classic symptoms of RSD include undue pain, skin sensitivity, coolness or warmth of the affected part, and mottling of the skin whereby it takes on a marble-like pattern. Not all of these symptoms and findings are present in every patient, and in some cases undue pain is the only abnormality.

NEUROMAS

Fine nerves as thin as a hair supply the sensation to your skin. These can become irritated by the surgery and lead to persistent pain in the area supplied by whatever nerves are irritated. So people who develop pain from neuromas are suffering from a skin—not a joint—condition!

NEUROPATHY

A *neuropathy* is a disease of one or more nerves. Diabetes, for example, can lead to a neuropathy, as can viruses, poisoning, and syphilis. A neuropathy will cause burning, numbness, and/or tingling in the part of the body supplied by the involved nerve.

It's been a matter of controversy whether *allergy* to a component of a metallic implant can cause loosening of an implant and/or pain. So far it has not been possible to accurately test for metal allergy. Just because you have some skin allergy to nickel, for example, does not automatically mean that you will be sensitive to the small amounts of nickel in a hip replacement. Conversely, the absence of any metal allergy in your medical history does not rule out the possibility of some allergy to your implant. As of this writing, there is no test to accurately tell if your hip or knee pain is the result of an allergy. The good news, however, is that such an allergy is (currently) considered to be rare.

> **Pain is transmitted by nerves. If the nerves themselves are "sick," a person feels pain.**

LACK OF PATELLA RESURFACING

Now we're getting technical. As we learned in chapter 14, the surgeon performing a knee replacement may or may not "resurface" the kneecap. Resurfacing the kneecap means removing the cartilage under the kneecap along with some bone, and replacing it with plastic. If you've not had the kneecap replaced, if your pain is very localized to the front of your knee, and if it's clear that the pain is not coming from one of the sources listed above, then your knee pain may be related to the absence of resurfacing. The cure for this is to have your surgeon resurface your kneecap. Because the tissues are stiff and leathery as a result of the first operation, the operation is more challenging the second time around. Moreover, in some patients, the pain persists.

NUMBNESS

Surgeons will discuss the more serious complications prior to your surgery, and leave out the more minor ones. There just isn't time. One of these "minor" issues doesn't feel so minor to a patient who is otherwise doing well and who hasn't been forewarned: More so after knee replacement than after hip replacement surgery, you might notice that the skin is numb. The numbness is mostly localized to the right side of the incision of a right knee and to the left side of the incision on a left knee replacement. This relates directly to the pattern of nerves supplying the sensation to the skin around your knee: Much of the sensation is derived from the saphenous nerve, which fans out into small branches across the front of the knee from left to right on a right knee and from right to left on a left knee. An incision down the front of the knee as is commonly used during knee replacement surgery interrupts those nerves. Thus a pattern of numbness to the outside of such incisions. These tiny nerves can slowly grow back over a period of months or years, allowing the numbness to resolve. It does not always completely resolve, however, and can be a cause of unhappiness. Fortunately, most patients will gladly trade in their knee pain for an area of numbness, and although patients not uncommonly bring up the subject, it is rarely a source of major dis-

> **After knee surgery, it is common for a person to note numbness to the outside of the incision.**

satisfaction (especially once they realize that it is not the result of a surgical error).

LEG LENGTHENING

This is a complication of hip replacement surgery much more so than of knee replacement surgery. It is referred to as *leg length discrepancy.*

Most patients readily adapt to the slight lengthening, considering it a small price to pay for the pain relief they have obtained.

Keep in mind that measuring leg lengths is an imprecise science. For any number of reasons, a surgeon may consciously or unconsciously over- or underestimate a patient's leg length discrepancy.

A certain amount of lengthening is normal, and I refer you to chapter 8 for a full discussion of the subject.

DISLOCATION

This topic has been addressed in chapters 8, 10, and 11, but it bears another short discussion. The "dislocation" complication pertains mainly to hip replacement surgery and refers to the ball popping out of the socket. This is a sudden and painful event. Every surgeon who performs hip replacement surgery is aware of this complication and during the surgery will do everything in his power to minimize the risk of a dislocation. The patient, in turn, can minimize the risks by avoiding certain maneuvers. The specific maneuvers to avoid depend on the surgical approach used by the surgeon to get to the hip (see chapter 8).

Make sure that by the time you leave the hospital, you clearly understand how to avoid these dangerous maneuvers.

When a surgeon dislocates a hip at the time of surgery, he first carefully dissects the tissues that surround the hip joint. When an *unexpected* dislocation occurs after surgery, however, those same tissues are violently torn. They don't heal as readily as they did following the surgery, and the patient is at a particular risk for another dislocation, especially in the first three months after the dislocation.

Should you suffer a dislocation, the surgeon may recommend a special brace. Hip braces are universally hated by patients and their use is controversial. We are in the process of developing a more patient-friendly brace, but the best course is to avoid a dislocation in the first place.

LOOSENING AND WEAR

A hip or knee replacement is a mechanical device, and like any mechanical device, it can loosen or wear out in time. When that happens, the patient often notes pain about the joint. The only treatment is to replace the implant. This is called *revision* surgery. This is often slow, risky, stressful surgery that no surgeon looks forward to. To make matters worse, in the United States if the patient is over the age of sixty-five, the surgeon will be reimbursed very poorly for his efforts (see chapter 20). All efforts are, therefore, geared toward creating systems that will last a patient's lifetime.

Loosening of the implant is sometimes visible on the X-ray: the implant will be noted to have shifted position when compared to the last X-ray, or a so-called lucency will have appeared between the implant and the bone. This lucency is an apparent space between the implant and the bone. Sometimes the lucency merely represents bone that is less dense and is of no concern, but if the lucency appears for the first time, it represents an empty space and indicates that the implant is no longer solidly anchored to the bone.

At the time of revision surgery, the loosening may not be visible to the naked eye. The surgeon might pull and twist the implant and not get it to budge, let alone remove it with his hands. The implant is said to be subject to *micromotion,* whereby motion takes place only when the patient puts his or her entire weight on the leg, and the motion that ensues between the implant and the surrounding bone is minuscule— but enough to cause pain.

How long does an implant last? Anywhere from a couple of years to thirty years or more. It depends on the design of the implant, the material that the implant is made of, the surgical technique, the activity of the patient, and yes, luck. (see chapter 19).

FOOT DROP, AKA DROP FOOT, PERONEAL NERVE PALSY

Who hasn't crossed their legs and had the top one "fall asleep"? This is because one of the main nerves supplying the foot, the *peroneal nerve,* runs close to the skin at the level of the knee. It is relatively easily compressed, and irritating it for any period of time will lead to numbness and tingling. The peroneal nerve is responsible for certain motions of the foot and ankle, and when compressed long enough, it stops working. In the mildest cases, a person will notice only weakness of the big toe, but in full-blown cases, the foot droops down and in (toward the midline). This makes it difficult to walk as the front of the foot catches the ground and causes the patient to stumble. Patients suffering from a foot drop, therefore, require an orthosis, a device that slips into a shoe. In this particular case, the orthosis is L-shaped with one branch of the L hugging the back of the lower calf. This is a reasonably cosmetic device, especially in someone wearing long pants, but the necessity of wearing one usually comes as an unpleasant surprise.

So why would a patient develop a foot drop after hip or knee replacement surgery?

The peroneal nerve is a branch of the sciatic nerve, which begins in the buttock area and runs behind the hip joint, down the back of the thigh, and into the lower leg. The specific point at which the peroneal nerve branches off from the sciatic nerve varies from person to person, but is generally located in the area of the hip joint. In theory, then, the sciatic nerve and/or its peroneal branch can be injured during a hip replacement. The injury can come in the form of direct compression from one of the somewhat pointy retractors used around the acetabulum to provide the surgeon with adequate exposure (see chapters 7 and 8). This is somewhat unusual because every hip surgeon is aware of this sciatic nerve and will adjust his technique accordingly (for example, I don't use any kind of pointy retractor in this area). The sciatic and peroneal nerves can also be injured from the simple *stretching* that occurs as the leg is maneuvered to and fro during the procedure. This is a particu-

> **A foot drop can occur in the absence of any wrongdoing. It seems to be more common in patients who have sustained a hip fracture.**

larly true in revision (redo) surgery when scarring of the tissues reduces their elasticity.

Patients who undergo hip replacement surgery for a hip fracture seem to be at greater risk for this complication. This is presumably because a fracture causes bleeding around the hip and because patients suffering from a hip fracture typically lie down for a prolonged period of time without moving—first on the ground, then in the emergency room, and then in the hospital bed. Thus, even prior to surgery, the sciatic and peroneal nerves have been compressed. The normal stretching that occurs during hip replacement surgery puts them over the top, and they wake up with a foot drop.

When did the foot drop occur? This question comes up rather frequently, especially when the foot drop is not noticed until a day or two after surgery. The question then arises as to whether the problem occurred during or after the surgery. We've just discussed how the peroneal nerve might be injured in the surgical suite. After the surgery, the straps that keep the foam pillow between your legs can also injure the peroneal nerve. Nurses in the recovery room occasionally perform a neurological evaluation by checking whether a patient can wiggle his or her toes. Since you can wiggle your toes even if your peroneal nerve is completely nonfunctional, a foot drop can be missed by such a perfunctory examination. Floor nurses or residents early on in their training can make the same mistake. Fortunately, the question is usually academic, meaning that the specific timing of the foot drop will not affect the recovery or treatment.

And by the way, one tests the peroneal nerve by checking the patient's ability to bring the ankle and toes toward the head (the opposite of letting the foot drop).

A foot drop can resolve over time. After six to twelve weeks the doctor may order a test called an EMG, which stands for electromyography. It's similar to having acupuncture, but not as much fun. The EMG can give your doctor an idea of exactly what nerve is affected, at what location it's been compromised, and what the prognosis (eventual outcome) might be.

The peroneal nerve is nowhere near the surgical site during a knee replacement. It is, therefore, very unlikely to be injured by any instrument. The nerve, however, can be stretched if the knee was deformed prior to the surgery and is straightened during the reconstruction. This is particularly true in the case of severe deformities. There are subtler causes of peroneal nerve palsy and they fall into the 2 + 2 = 5 category. A patient will have spinal stenosis, for example. This is a spinal condition where the space for the spinal cord narrows and squeezes the nerves exiting the spine. The patient may be totally asymptomatic, meaning that he or she is completely unaware of this condition. This same patient now undergoes a knee replacement during which time a tourniquet is applied to the leg. This may also compromise the function of the peroneal nerve (nerves need blood too!). Upon recovering from anesthesia, a foot drop is noted.

Note that foot drops after knee replacement surgery performed in the absence of a significant deformity are distinctly rare.

NERVE INJURIES

We've just discussed peroneal nerve palsies, and prior to that we discussed the numbness that is associated with the division of small sensory nerves under the skin. That leaves us with just the *femoral nerve*. This is a major nerve that supplies the quadriceps muscles at the front of the thigh. It runs in front of the acetabulum and is invisible during a hip replacement operation. It is extremely unlikely to be injured, but in a difficult case a retractor placed too far from the acetabulum could place undue pressure on the nerve.

VASCULAR INJURIES

Major blood vessels course about the hip and knee. Remarkably, then, vascular injuries are rare.

The hip. Directly behind the acetabulum where the cup is to be placed (see chapters 7 and 8) lie the *iliac artery* and *vein*, major vessels that course toward the leg. These vessels are at risk when the surgeon uses screws to help fix the cup to the bone. Fortunately, the location of the iliac artery and vein is constant, and is known to every hip surgeon. Problems arise when the acetabulum is deformed and the surgeon is obligated to place a screw from an unusual location or angle. Even more unusual, a surgeon may be called upon to remove a cup that has migrated into the pelvis (yes, *migrated* is the technical term). The cup may have melded with the iliac vein or artery, and upon its removal one or both vessels are injured. When the surgeon suspects such a scenario, he often calls upon a vascular surgeon to dissect the artery and vein from the cup prior to removing the cup. Again, let me emphasize that this is not an issue during a primary (first-time) hip replacement![1]

When the surgeon is preparing the other half of the total hip replacement, namely, the femur (thighbone), major vessels

1. First time for the patient, that is.

are even less at risk, especially if the orthopedist is approaching the hip from the lateral side (where the opening to your pants pocket is). Indeed, the major artery and vein in the neighborhood—the *femoral artery* and *vein*—lie at the front of the thigh. Nevertheless, many of their tributaries are around the hip, some of which must be divided for the surgeon to gain access to the hip joint. In the average patient, these vessels are easily clamped and coagulated. In the occasional patient, the slightest little vessel bleeds continuously. This hampers visibility, wears on the surgeon's patience, and leads to greater-than-average blood loss. For this reason, the surgeon will urge you to stay away from medications that diminish blood clotting such as aspirin (see chapter 5).

The knee. There are two sets of blood vessels about the knee. The *geniculate arteries* and *veins* run about the sides and front of the knee and tend to be small. But there are many of them, their exact location varies from patient to patient, and one or more must be sectioned off during a total knee replacement. They account for all of the bleeding that occurs during and after a routine knee replacement. Fortunately, with a little patience the surgeon can coagulate the vessels and limit the blood loss. He cannot control 100 percent of the blood loss, however, which is why a person's blood count will often drop in the two days or so following surgery.

Of greater concern are the femoral artery and vein—the same structures that course at the front of the hip. Fortunately for the knee surgeon, these vessels now find themselves at the *back* of the knee. Retractors keep the artery and nerve out of harm's way. Most of the time. In fact, essentially all of the time. It is true that the surgeon is using a power saw from front to back as he removes a sliver of bone from the upper tibia (shinbone), and an element of risk always remains. If for whatever reason the artery or vein lies in an unusual location, the saw can snag the vessel. This is not a subtle complication, as the bleeding is usually impressive. A vascular surgeon must be called in to address the injury. The greatest challenge comes when the vessel is *completely* transected, causing the vessel to immediately go into spasm and retract into the thigh: There is no bleeding to suggest a vascular injury! To keep things in perspective, note that most knee surgeons will never see this in their lifetime. Vascular injuries about the hip and knee are rare. If you want something realistic to be concerned about, worry about knee stiffness. At least it's something you have control over.

SUMMARY

Total hip and total knee replacement operations are truly one of God's gifts to humankind. Countless suffering folk have been given a new life thanks to these operations. But of course, there are risks, and the purpose of this chapter has been to lay these on the line. Keep in mind, however, that these risks are relatively rare; otherwise, joint replacement surgery wouldn't still be so popular. If you've been burdened with intractable pain for a long time and you are reasonably healthy, you should undergo the surgery.

Chapter 19

❧

Do You Really Want the Latest Implant? The Mini-Incision, Partial Knee Spacers, and Other Controversies

As a consumer, you are used to getting the latest. The latest car, the latest tennis racquet, the latest MP3. So naturally you'll want the latest hip or knee replacement.

Or will you?

Improvements in auto mechanics and MP3 technology ensure you that each new model will indeed reflect a higher level of performance than the previous one. Now look at the history of hip and knee implants: The orthopedic highway is littered with implants that "seemed like a good idea at the time."

They appear with a flourish, supported by extensive advertising and sometimes ballyhooed by the media—and disappear.

Surgeons who specialize in joint replacements are faced with a very unique problem: They have to wait fifteen to twenty-five years to see if their products are any better than the previous ones. You see, there are hip and knee replacements that already last that long. Yes, extensive testing is carried out.

The FDA is a strict, powerful institution that places remarkable demands on implant manufacturers. No amount of testing, however, duplicates the stresses placed upon an implant imbedded in the human body for decades on end.

> A joint replacement is not a car. Despite the hype, not every "advance" turns out to be a true improvement.

The history of the plastic used in joint replacement surgery is illustrative. Many plastic-like materials were tried before Sir John Charnley in England happened upon ultra-high molecular weight polyethylene (UHMWPE). Other materials wore out too quickly or elicited a nasty biological reaction (Teflon being such a material). UHMWPE has served humanity well. Millions of people have walked the Earth pain-free thanks to implant linings made of this material.

But it isn't perfect.

Over time it slowly wears out. More significantly it wears out at an unpredictable rate (see chapter 18). Multiple attempts have, therefore, been made at improving the already excellent wear properties of UHMWPE. Each new "improvement" has been extensively tested. Yet at least two products based on these "improvements" have worn out even faster than the original.

When the orthopedic industry introduced cementless cups (see chapter 8), it was to improve upon the durability of the all-plastic cups that were cemented into position. Some of the models lasted far less long than the all-plastic cups.

Someone had the clever idea that cups could be designed

with threads so as to be literally screwed into the pelvis. The idea caught on and was very popular in the mid- to late 1980s. Now go ahead, ask your orthopedist whether screw-in cups are still part of his armamentarium (they are not).

Titanium alloys were introduced in the 1980s. Hip stems made of this material have just a little more flexibility than steel or cobalt-chrome stems, a feature felt by some to be desirable. The femoral ball that snaps on to these stems was also switched to titanium to match the material of

> **The plastic bearing is made of very tough polyethylene. Nevertheless, over time it slowly wears down. The orthopedic industry has consistently tried to improve upon it.**

the stem. A few thousand patients later, it was discovered that these titanium heads were wearing down. It turns out that titanium does not make for a very good "bearing" material because it is too soft. Many patients who received these titanium femoral heads then needed further surgery to replace them.

So here is the point: If there already exists a technique and an implant that is likely to provide you with lasting pain relief and acceptable function, think twice about asking for or accepting an implant with no track record.

There is always room for improvement, and new products are always being brought to market. Do *you* want to be the pio-

> **Are you interested in being a pioneer? Great! Make sure you know what you're getting into!**

neer who will test these out? Maybe yes. We do need such people, and if you are one of them, God bless you. You should do so, however, as an informed consumer.

Here are some of the newer products and my thoughts about them.

COMPUTER-GUIDED HIP REPLACEMENTS

Thumbs-up. To avoid dislocation of a hip replacement, the surgeon must position the cup within a certain range of angles. This alone does not guarantee a stable hip, but it's a start. Unfortunately, positioning the cup is not as precise a science as it could be. There are a number of reasons for this, such as the variable positioning of the patient on the operating table. Some form of computer-assisted guidance will be a welcome addition, unless femoral head sizes can be safely increased to the point where the risk of dislocation becomes negligible (see chapters 8, 10, 11, and 18).

HIP REPLACEMENTS PERFORMED THROUGH MINI-INCISIONS

Thumbs-up, thumbs-down.

The term *mini-incision* is used to describe two different operations: the traditional hip replacement performed through a smaller-than-usual incision, and a hip replacement performed through *two* even smaller incisions.

I give an unqualified thumbs-up to the first of these two mini-incisions. Traditional hip incisions, which usually run about six inches or more, are often much longer than they need to be. Keep in mind that the larger the leg and the more challenging the case, the longer the incision needs to be for the surgeon to see what he is doing.

As for the second type of mini-incision, I give it thumbs-down—for now. Note that I said "for now." Things change, and this technique may turn out to be terrific. Right now it's very much in the developmental stages. Here's how it works: Two smaller incisions, each about two to three inches long, replace the standard skin incision. One incision is "posterior" to the standard incision (closer to the buttock), and the other is anterior (farther from the buttock) to the standard incision. The surgeon can no longer consistently look directly into your hip joint. In order to see what he is doing, the surgeon relies on a serious amount of fluoroscopy (X-rays) throughout the procedure.

Here are the problems I anticipate: A total joint replacement can be a straightforward procedure, but it can also be tricky. Sometimes the surgeon can differentiate between the two ahead of time; sometimes he notes a little surprise at the time of surgery.

For the thin, straightforward patient, just about any approach will work.

In the case of the patient with a large thigh and/or an unusual hip joint, the prudent surgeon will know ahead of time not to recommend small incisions.

The real problem occurs with the borderline patient. The premise (and promise) of a small incision may be why you selected your surgeon in the first place. If the surgeon uses anything but the mini-incision, he hasn't delivered on his promise, or at least his *implied* promise. So the surgeon who is committed to the mini-incision sees it as a loss of face to switch to a standard incision in the middle of an operation. He perseveres with the mini-incision and you end up with a complication or a less-than-optimal result.

The two-incision, X-ray-guided hip replacement poses a

particular problem: The operation is radically different from what your surgeon has been trained to do. His visualization is greatly diminished and he must compensate for this by relying on crude, two-dimensional, black-and-white shadows (X-rays). Since we are still in the very early stages of this approach, expect to see a slew of complications early on. Ideally you'd want to wait ten years to see if the long-term results are as good as those obtained with traditional replacements. No one is going to want to wait that long. At least wait five years, however, to see how the short- and medium-term complications shake out.

> **Remember: Patients undergoing hip replacement surgery by way of standard incisions heal well and quickly. There are no studies showing that replacements placed through two tiny incisions are placed accurately or securely. It will take a few years to prove or disprove this.**

The standard hip replacement does not cut any major muscle.

Finally, the size of the skin incision is not the major determinant of a patient's recovery.

So while the surgeon should seriously think of cutting down on the length of the standard hip incision, it's a very serious error for either the surgeon or the patient to make this the number one priority. Your main focus should be on obtaining a pain- and trouble-free hip replacement that will last you a lifetime.

TOTAL KNEE REPLACEMENTS PERFORMED THROUGH MINI-INCISIONS

Maybe yes. This already makes more sense to me because the length of the traditional incision and the surgical dissection do have a direct impact on recovery. Smaller incisions and surgical approaches that do not involve flipping over the kneecap offer a realistic expectation of a quicker recovery. On the other hand, this type of surgery is also in its early, early infancy, and it is even harder to perform a complete knee replacement through a small incision than a hip replacement. My feeling is that you are going to find a high rate of complications associated with this small-incision total knee replacement surgery until all the kinks have been worked out and specific criteria are established for who should and who shouldn't undergo such surgery. For now, I'd stay away unless you are the direct descendant of Lewis and Clark and the pioneering spirit runs through your veins.

PARTIAL KNEE REPLACEMENTS PERFORMED THROUGH MINI-INCISIONS

Thumbs-up. Partial knee replacements have traditionally been implanted through a standard total knee replacement incision. It is now pretty clear that these small implants can be introduced by way of a much smaller incision. Perhaps not "mini," but at least half as much as the traditional incision.

KNEE "SPACERS"

Thumbs-down. The concept of inserting "knee spacers" is appealing (and over forty years old). If the cartilage in part of the knee has worn out, just put something in there to fill the missing space. The "Uni spacer" places a metal disk that is flat on one side and concave on the other. It comes in different sizes, the idea being that if precisely the right size is chosen, this free-floating disk will stay put and provide pain relief. Crazier ideas have worked but I'm not going to be standing at the front of the line for this one. It's hard for me to imagine that a piece of metal wedged into a knee is going to provide pain relief on a consistent basis. A regular joint replacement that moves ever so slightly when you stand up is quite painful, so it's hard to imagine that this spacer won't be. Maybe I'll turn out to be wrong on this one, too. I'd wait for some results to come in.

CERAMIC-ON-CERAMIC HIP REPLACEMENTS

One thumb up. In a ceramic-on-ceramic hip replacement, the plastic UHMWPE liner that snaps into the metal shell is replaced by a ceramic liner. The femoral head is also made of ceramic. Ceramic articulating (rubbing) against ceramic exhibits lower friction than metal on plastic or ceramic on plastic. This leads to less wear of the liner and possibly to a longer-lasting implant. Because of the limited wear, the surgeon can use a larger femoral head, which in turn tends to decrease the risk of dislocation (see chapters 8 and 18). On the other hand, the ceramic doesn't allow for a protective lip around the back of the cup as does a plastic liner, and this may *increase* the risk of dislocation. The two factors probably cancel out except in very large patients, where the surgeon can implant a truly large femoral head. Ceramic-on-ceramic hip replacements have been available in Europe for over twenty years, but have just recently been cautiously introduced in the United States. They are very expensive and in some ways are fragile. For now they are reserved for the young, active, and/or heavy patient.

It is important to note that ceramics represent an entire class of materials. Although all ceramics share certain properties (hardness, smoothness, brittleness, improved lubrication, lower friction), not all ceramics are equally suited for joint replacement surgery. Alumina and zirconia are two ceramics that have been used for many years.

METAL-ON-METAL HIP REPLACEMENTS

One thumb up. This is an old idea that has been recently resurrected. As with the ceramic-ceramic hip, the surgeon does away with the UHMWPE altogether. A metallic head articulates against a thin metal liner (figure 19.1). When first tried forty years ago, it was not successful. The design of the implants was poor and metallic debris was found scattered all over the hip joint. In its latest incarnation, however, the metal ball and cup are machined so precisely that a fine fluid film continuously lubricates every part of the articulation. Relatively few visible metallic particles are released. For technical reasons, a metal liner can be much thinner than a plastic one. This means that the femoral head can be larger (even larger than a ceramic femoral head), and this diminishes the risk of dislocation after surgery (see chapters 8 and 18).

Metal-on-metal hip replacements are expensive and, as

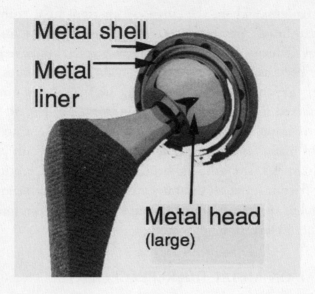

Figure 19.1. "Metal on metal" total hip replacement. *(Courtesy DePuy Orthopaedics, Inc.)*

with the ceramic-ceramic implants, they are currently reserved for the young, heavy, active patient.

SUMMARY

Every year you will hear of new implants and new techniques. If the past is any predictor of the future, most novelties will disappear. A few thousand brave or naïve patients will pay the price for these failures. On the other hand, after a few hiccups for which some patients will also pay, certain innovations will turn out to be true improvements and will change the face of joint replacement surgery. Patients who will have been in on these improvements in their early phase will look back proudly on their bravery and good fortune.

Are you ready to roll the dice?

Chapter 20

❊❊

The Economics of
Joint Replacement Surgery

There are as many brands of hip and knee replacements as there are automobiles. Your surgeon assesses your case carefully and scans the implant horizon to pick the replacement that's just right for you.

Dream on.

It should not come as a great shock to you to find that decisions made about your joint replacement surgery are dictated in part by financial considerations. Before you start sweating, the good news is that your well-being is not seriously threatened. American orthopedic surgeons are well trained, and joint replacement implants are manufactured and tested in a sound way. But financial considerations are never far from the surface.

First of all, you should know that Medicare and HMOs don't take joint replacement surgery very seriously—at least not judged by what they pay surgeons. Whereas they will readily pay for unnecessary knee MRIs and knee arthroscopies (see

What Your Doctor May Not *Tell You about Knee Pain and Surgery*, Warner Books, 2002), they cry poverty when it comes to your joint replacement. The the New York city Medicare reimbursement for a hip replacement is around $1,800 and is heading south. This fee includes not only the surgery but also three months of follow-up visits and phone calls. The reimbursement for a knee replacement is even lower. Add up the hours and divide into 1,800 or 1,600 and . . . well, I won't go there, it's too depressing. Keep in mind the fact that a healthy chunk of the surgeon's payment has to be earmarked to his $75,000 to $100,000 (or more) yearly insurance premium. The point is that if Medicare or an HMO is paying your "in network" surgeon, he's not making much money off your surgery. He's performing the surgery because he enjoys it, because he's good at it, because he cares for you, and/or because he's got an operating room slot to fill.

> **HMOs and Medicare don't seem to mind shelling out millions of dollars for unnecessary MRIs and arthroscopies, but they'll pay your joint replacement surgeon only rock-bottom fees.**

Here's something for you to consider: The surgeon receives the same payment whether the surgery is easy or complicated, whether the surgery is short or long, whether he takes a short cut or goes the extra mile. Let's see how that might color his judgment: Suppose that your hip anatomy is very different from that of the average person. Your surgeon considers a surgical approach that involves removing a piece of the thighbone at the beginning of the surgery and placing it back at the end of the procedure (a surgical approach called a *trochanteric osteotomy*). This adds time, complexity, and potential short-term complications to the procedure, but it leads to a sounder hip replacement. The surgeon is not going to receive an extra dime for this trochanteric osteotomy.

A more common scenario is that faced by the knee surgeon on a weekly basis: When performing a total knee replacement, the surgeon can resurface the kneecap or not (see chapter 14). In other words, he can just leave it alone or take the time to remove some cartilage and bone and replace them with a plastic implant (*resurfacing*). Resurfacing will add time to the operation. Not a dollar, not a penny, not a Euro, not a ruble more can the surgeon expect for taking this extra time. So guess what? Studies have been undertaken to prove that resurfacing the kneecap is not necessary. Not all studies have led to this conclusion, but your surgeon has ample ammunition to back him up when he decides to leave your kneecap untouched. I myself have gone back and forth on this issue and now decide what to do on a case-by-case basis.

> If your surgeon goes the extra mile, he won't see an extra penny.

Let us say you have arthritis in just the inner (medial) compartment of your knee. Let us also assume that your surgeon is hesitating between a partial (unicompartmental) and a total knee replacement (see chapter 14). The partial replacement is as hard or harder to implant than the total replacement. Medicare and private insurance companies, however, see this partial replacement as "half" a total knee replacement—and pay half. Considering that there are valid arguments for using either implant, the surgeon with no particular interest in partial replacements will pick the total knee replacement.

In certain parts of the world the situation is reversed. The surgeon is given a budget for the year. He can spend just so much money on his knee implants. The partial replacements cost less than the total replacements, and by using the partial implants the surgeon can treat more patients. He will be far more inclined to choose the partial replacement.

When a new implant hits the market, you figure that it's been extensively tested. Yes and no. Serious engineers have studied it into the wee hours of the night and it's been extensively tested *in the lab*. No amount of testing, however, can tell you what specifically will happen when the joint replacement is implanted into the human body. Imagine, for instance, that the Acme Company has an idea for a new metal rod to be used for the fixation of femur fractures. The success of that rod will depend on its ease of insertion, its versatility, and its ability to hold the fracture fragments together until they heal. A fracture heals within three to six months, so the Acme Company will know in short order whether their new product marks a true improvement in the field of fracture surgery.

> **In the United States a surgeon is financially disinclined to use a partial knee replacement. In other parts of the world the opposite is true.**

Now imagine instead that the Acme Company has an idea for a new hip or knee replacement designed to be more durable. Today's implants last at least ten years if not twenty, so Acme will have to wait at least that long to see if their product is truly better. There is also the chance that their implant will be inferior despite the extensive bench work that has been performed. Their implant, for example, may last only eight years. The logical approach would, therefore, be to implant the new replacement in a relatively small number of patients who would be observed a minimum of ten years. If the new replacement were found to be at least as durable as the existing ones, it could then be safely released for the general public.

No dice.

No manufacturer can afford to wait for ten years of clinical trials before releasing a product. The general public becomes the test market. This gets us back to the point that I made in the last chapter about not automatically rushing to the front of the line when a new implant comes out.

> **No manufacturer can afford to do the right thing: wait ten to twenty years to see if a new hip or knee replacement is at least as good as current models.**

You would think that your doctor's reimbursement for a given operation would be somewhat proportional to the length, complexity, medical risks, and medico-legal risks involved. Not so. In fact, it's quite the reverse.

Relatively speaking, a short, low-risk operation such as an arthroscopy is reimbursed at a reasonable rate. A hip or knee replacement pays poorly. A revision (redo) replacement, one of the most tedious, time-consuming, labor-intensive, and risky operations in all of surgery pays worst of all.

Insurance companies will sometimes reimburse surgeons according to the nature of the condition, not the nature of the surgery. For example, an orthopedist who provides you with a total hip replacement because you broke your hip will be paid far less than the orthopedist in the operating room next door performing the exact same procedure on a patient suffering from hip arthritis! The surgeon who is hesitating between a total and a partial hip replacement in a patient with a hip fracture is consequently *financially* disinclined to choose the total replacement (which is not to say that he won't do so out of your best interest). If Medicare is footing the bill, the surgeon is not allowed to ask the patient for any form of extra compensation nor is the patient even allowed to do so of his or her own free will. The subject will, therefore, never come up in your discussion with the surgeon—but he's thinking about it, I guarantee you!

Consider your preoperative evaluation. This is where you go to your family doctor for him or her to evaluate your overall medical health. Your doctor will want to perform basic blood tests, a cardiogram, and a chest X-ray unless they've been recently done. If any abnormalities are detected, your doctor may want to repeat this or that test. If you suffer from a medical condition—say coronary heart disease—your doctor will want the advice of a specialist, in this case a cardiologist. The cardiologist will, in turn, order one or more tests. Your medical doctor may need to see you a second time. Needless to say, it is a good idea to start this process a few weeks before the surgery so as not to run out of time as the day

> **Your surgery may get canceled at the last minute because your insurance doesn't pay for timely preoperative evaluations.**

of surgery approaches. A peaceful and timely preoperative evaluation ensures that when you go for that final evaluation at the hospital's preadmission testing, there won't be any surprises. This has been the traditional modus operandi.

More and more, though, the preoperative evaluation is all

packed into the week before surgery and the hospital's preadmission testing results are used as the basis for the evaluation. The outcome of this approach is obvious: Every now and then surgeries are canceled at the last moment. The sand has run out of the hourglass before questionable results could be checked out.

The reason for this shift in attitude has everything to do with dollars and cents. Your family doctor can't be sure that he or she will get paid for the peaceful, prudent approach. If it's something you feel you might afford, find out from your doctor what it would cost you out of pocket to schedule a preliminary visit a few weeks before surgery.

Chapter 21

❦

How to Choose a Surgeon[1]

Y ou want the best surgeon around. Who wants the second best? Fortunately there are many *best* surgeons around. You want a surgeon with experience and one with whom you feel comfortable. You are building a long-term relationship. Contrary to the surgeon who takes out your appendix or gallbladder, your joint replacement surgeon will be following you on a regular basis for an indefinite period of time. If problems develop, will he be there for you?

> You want the best surgeon around. Who wants the second best?

You are looking for the right combination of technical ability and personality.

Your options include:

1. The orthopedic surgeon nearest you.

---

1. This has been adapted from *What Your Doctor May Not Tell You About Knee Pain and Surgery*, Warner Books, 2002.

2. The orthopedic surgeon with the biggest ad in the phone book or the most impressive Web site.

3. The orthopedic surgeon referred by a friend or a coworker.

4. The team orthopedic surgeon for your favorite professional sports team.

5. The orthopedic surgeon referred by your family physician.

6. An orthopedic surgeon taken from the list of board-certified M.D.s, provided by a state medical society or by the American Academy of Orthopaedic Surgeons.

7. The orthopedic surgeon recommended by a hospital's referral service.

8. An orthopedic surgeon listed in *The Best Doctors in . . . [Your City]*.

9. A doctor referred by a nurse, a resident in training, or an administrator at a hospital.

10. An orthopedic surgeon with an impressive résumé.

11. A department chairman.

12. A doctor referred by another orthopedist.

Each of these has merit, yet one stands out as being better than all others. Let us look at each individually:

The doctor nearest you. Obviously, by simply going to the doctor nearest you, you are taking a major gamble. This requires no explanation.

The doctor with the biggest ad in the phone book or the most impressive Web site. Most savvy customers will know not to be impressed by an advertisement in the phone book. A large ad merely reflects the doctor's willingness to spend money on promotion. This is often effective since most of the population is not savvy. Educated customers, though, can still be taken in by Web page promotions. It is important to keep in mind that a doctor can make any claim on his or her home page. A health professional can pay to have an *entire textbook* on the Web! It doesn't mean that the health professional actually knows everything in that book or has even read it!

The Web is merely the phone book of the new millennium.

The doctor referred by a friend or a coworker. A doctor recommendation from a friend, relative, or coworker is fairly frequent. Everybody goes to the best doctor in town and people freely dispense advice. Such a recommendation tells you that at least *someone* has gotten better under that doctor's care—but it doesn't tell you if it was thanks to, or in spite of, the surgeon. It also doesn't tell you about the doctor's ethics or knowledge of your particular problem. An orthopedist who was great at treating your buddy's back pain may not be so hot when it comes to performing joint replacements.

The team doctor for your favorite professional sports team. There's a reason why hospitals will pay professional teams a million dollars and up to have one of their docs be the team orthopedist: Being a team doctor is a terrific draw. And no book that anybody writes is going to change this. The thinking among the public is, "If he's good enough for the Jersey Jupiters, he's good enough for me." Having said this, is he good enough for the Jupiters? Sometimes yes, sometimes no. There are some very knowledgeable and ethical team doctors and some, well, not so ethical. The position of team doctor is not always won on merit. Also, by and large, joint replacement surgery is not the specialty of team orthopedists. Chances are you will be referred to one of the team doctor's colleagues.

The doctor referred by your family physician. One thing that can be said for your family physician is that he or she has your best interests in mind—which is a start. Not all family physicians, though, recognize the intricacies of orthopedics to the point of differentiating between orthopedists who are particularly strong in one area versus those who are strong in another area. Ask your doctor if he or she would recommend the same orthopedist whether you had back or knee pain.

A doctor taken from the list of board-certified M.D.s, provided by a state medical society or by the American Academy of Orthopaedic Surgeons. "Board certification" is not a bad thing. If an orthopedist has been certified at some point by the American Board of Orthopaedic Surgery, it tells the potential customer that the surgeon has trained in an accredited American program and that he or she has studied hard to pass a written and oral examination. But in the setting of joint replacement surgery, board certification is not as important as it might seem. The board certification examination covers an enormously wide range of subjects, including dwarfism, metallurgy, muscle physiology, cartilage biochemistry, wheelchair principles, and prosthetic limbs. Thrown in there, are a few broad questions on joint replacements. Moreover, board certification is no guarantee of technical ability. In short, board certification in and of itself is not a good selection criterion.

The doctor recommended by a hospital's referral service. All major hospitals have a referral service, usually with a catchy toll-free telephone number such as 1-877-COM TO US. They will never tell you, "We don't have anyone who performs joint replacements." Instead, they'll read you the names of orthopedists *who have listed themselves* as being interested in joint replacements or joint reconstruction. This, if you will, is the Yellow Pages of the hospital and just about as useful. You are better off contacting the orthopedic department directly, though here, the staff will have some allegiance to the chairman and to his or her inner circle.

A doctor listed in The Best Doctors in . . . [Your City]. There are a number of books purporting to give you a list of the best professionals around. Some are for real and some are bogus. Here's how the bogus ones work. Doctors are sent an application to fill out: name, address, specialty, etc. The doctors who take the time to complete the form are included in the directory. When the book comes out, who buys it? All the doctors listed, of course! Everybody wins: The doctors are listed in a prestigious-sounding text, the publishing company earns a profit from all the doctors who bought the book, and nobody can accuse the doctors of having paid to be listed. Well, almost everybody wins. Anybody leafing through such a book in search of the "best doctors" is rolling the dice.

Other directories make more of an effort to truly find the best doctors. Be aware that these are imperfect, too. Some excellent surgeons toil in relative obscurity. They may not publish or lecture much and, therefore, will remain unknown outside their hospital. Others will have recently moved to a new hospital and not have formed a "base" yet. Yet others are the shy, retiring type and will not attract any attention. This is somewhat rare for orthopedic surgeons, however.

Read the first pages of any *Best Doctors* book to see how the doctors were selected.

A doctor referred by a nurse, a resident in training, or an administrator at a hospital. A hospital staff sees hip and knee surgeons up close and personal. But few staff members see all the important aspects of a surgeon's practice. Nurses in the operating room get a sense of a surgeon's technical ability, but can't say much about bedside manner or a surgeon's indications for surgery. Floor nurses can tell you about bedside manner and postoperative attention to patients, but are less informed on technical ability and, again, surgical indications. Administrators can tell you which surgeons are busy, but can't tell you why they are busy. (Are they good doctors or just good salesmen?) Residents (surgeons in training) are a good source of information with regard to the surgeons at their particular hospital, especially if they have a chance to participate in that surgeon's office hours. Because they are in training, though, they may lack some perspective and are susceptible to being won over by charismatic surgeons and/or swell guys who let them do cases. They also lack the ability to compare their teachers to other surgeons in town.

A doctor with an impressive résumé. An impressive résumé tells you that the surgeon has given a great deal of thought to this area of study. If he is asked to lecture, he is probably thought of as being knowledgeable, and more significantly, if he has widely published, he probably has expertise in the area of his publications. A résumé, though, doesn't tell you about patient management and ethics.

A department chairman. The chairman of an orthopedic department is suave, debonair, good-looking, intelligent, and highly skilled,[2] and it is natural for patients to seek out the advice of such a doctor. Chairmen (chairwomen are quite rare) are chosen on the basis of their particular expertise in one area

2. My chairman could conceivably be reading this book.

of orthopedics and/or leadership and administrative skills. Their appreciation for the subtleties of the joint replacement ranges from excellent to minimal, depending on their area of expertise. Chairmen are usually surrounded by a well-organized staff and have the full attention of the senior orthopedic residents (residents in their last year of training). This may or may not compensate for the fact that some chairmen are away from their practice a great deal. Make sure this is not something that would bother you.

A doctor referred by another orthopedist. Bingo. A referral from an orthopedist is not easy to come by, unless you happen to be related to one or have one as a friend. (Everybody should!). Nevertheless, this is your best bet. You might even consider paying for a consultation just to get such a referral. Orthopedists know the orthopedic "salesmen" in their community as well as the guys with suspect ethics or poor bedside manner. They know this better than any layperson and, for obvious reasons, better than doctors in other specialties. The advice of an orthopedist is not foolproof, of course. If you live in a large community, no orthopedist will be familiar with the particular strengths and shortcomings of *all* his colleagues. If the orthopedist has something bad to say about the doctor you had in mind, it could be because of rivalries and jealousies. Conversely, an orthopedist may be interested in helping a friend. Nevertheless, it is unlikely that an orthopedist would let you make a big mistake.

In an ideal world, you would have access to all of the above options and they would all point to one or two knee doctors in your community. Realistically, you will have access to just a few of the options I have listed. My advice would be to use as many as possible.

Chapter 22

Answers to Common Questions

How do I know when I need a joint replacement?

When your pain becomes intractable despite all reasonable nonoperative approaches. You don't need a joint replacement just because the X-ray "looks bad."

Where do I find a surgeon who can put in a hip replacement through a mini-incision?

Go back to chapter 19 to find out why you are asking the wrong question. You want a surgeon who can give you a pain-free hip for a long time to come.

How long should my joint replacement last?

Ten years. At least that's the party line. Many implants will last over twenty years. After that either the implant loosens or the bearing wears out, especially if you are still young or active at that point.

Where is the hip joint?

Not where you think it is! The hip joint is closer to the front of your thigh than to your butt. A hip problem will, therefore, tend to cause pain in the groin area, at the crease between your upper thigh and belly. Pain in the area of your butt is much more likely to come from a pinched nerve in your back than from a hip problem.

Is arthritis always painful?

No! This is true of arthritis anywhere in the body. You can have arthritis for years without even knowing it. Don't let yourself get talked into a joint replacement on the basis of a "bad looking" X-ray. ("Mrs. Jones, this X-ray looks terrible. Why don't we replace your knee at the beginning of next month?")

Are some implants glued in?

No. There is no glue in joint replacement surgery. Many implants are cemented in place, but the cement isn't sticky. No more so than the cement between two bricks.

Is the whole knee removed in a *total* knee replacement?

No. Only slivers at the ends of the bone are removed.

What is a hip dislocation?

The hip joint consists of a ball and a socket. When the ball slips out of the socket, the hip is said to have dislocated. This is a painful situation. The process of putting it back in is called the *reduction*, and once the process is complete, the hip is said to be *reduced*.

Are there warning signs before a hip dislocates?

Alas, no. Heed the precautions taught to you by your surgeon, nurse, and therapist, and don't count on any warning signs. If your hip pops out, it will do so in a fraction of a second.

Is a hip dislocation a lifelong risk? Do I have to watch what I do the rest of my life?

Yes. After a while the precautions become second nature.

What's the big deal about a "revision" (redo) joint replacement?

Redoing a hip replacement is much more difficult and much riskier than a first-time replacement. This is true anywhere in the body, and it is the result of the tissues being much less soft and pliable. Also, dense scar will have wrapped itself around everything, and this will have to be slowly and methodically peeled away by the surgeon before he can do anything to your hip or knee.

Why the reluctance on the surgeon's part to place a joint replacement in a young person?

The implant will loosen or wear out in the person's lifetime, thus subjecting them to a revision.

I am eighty-two years old. Am I too old for a joint replacement?

It's a question of health and motivation, not age. In fact, there's no advantage to waiting. The implant will last your lifetime. If you meet all the criteria for a joint replacement, have the procedure while your doctor still allows it.

Why won't my doctor let me play tennis after a joint replacement?

He might let you play some easy doubles, but he'll discourage you from any vigorous running and twisting. Unless, of course, he doesn't plan on being around when you've worn out the bearing of your joint replacement and it needs to be replaced.

Can I get an MRI if I've had a joint replacement?

Yes. Your implant is metallic but nonmagnetic. The pictures produced by an MRI will be blurry in the immediate vicinity of the implant, but it is not dangerous to undergo an MRI. Pictures taken of areas away from the joint replacement will be perfectly clear.

Why do I need to see my surgeon on a regular basis even if I'm feeling well?

You won't feel the plastic wearing out in your joint replacement. If this should happen to any significant degree, the microscopic debris may cause the surrounding bone to gradually disappear. And you won't feel that either until a massive amount of bone is gone! Better to discover this early.

It's been three months and I'm still having pain after my joint replacement. Is this normal?

Not if the pain is severe. Some achiness is normal, but no more than that—especially in the hip. The knee can be sore from the bending and straightening exercises. In the first three months, pain can be attributed to the surgery itself, but after three months, the surgeon will start to look for other sources of pain.

I need a joint replacement and I've just read about a new type of implant. I should make sure my surgeon uses this model. Right or wrong?

Wrong. Your implant should last you ten, twenty, or thirty years, if not longer. If it hasn't been around that long, how do you know it will? Because of the manufacturer's assurances? Note that no manufacturer will ever make that assurance on a new implant. And most implants introduced since the inception of joint replacement surgery have not stood the test of time.

Joint replacement is big-time surgery and the surgeon is making big-time bucks. Right or Wrong?

Wrong. Although a surgeon may occasionally be well reimbursed, the average hip or knee replacement earns a surgeon between $1,600 and $1,800—and that includes three months of follow-up care no matter how stormy your postoperative course is. An orthopedic surgeon pays upwards of $75,000 a year in malpractice insurance. You do the math.

Will my implant set off the alarms at the airport?

It used to be unlikely, but since 9/11, the possibility of setting off an alarm has increased.

A special joint replacement ID card will allow me to breeze through airport security, no?

No. Anybody in the terror business can make an ID purporting to show that the bearer has had a joint replacement. No halfway competent airport security guard is going to wave you on just because you have an ID card.

In performing a hip replacement, is it not harmful to remove the marrow from the thighbone?

No. The marrow found in the upper femur (thighbone) doesn't produce blood cells in any significant quantity.

What is a "press-fit" implant?

An implant needs to be fixed to the underlying bone. If it is pressed/jammed/impacted into the bone rather than being cemented, it is said to be press-fit.

Should I have both hips/knees replaced on the same day?

Maybe. It's a lot of surgery. You have to be physically and mentally up to it. I usually recommend operating on one hip or knee at a time unless the other one is so bad that rehabilitation will be impossible. Your family doctor will have a say in this.

What's the difference between the *true* and *apparent* length of my leg, and why does it matter?

The apparent leg length is what you feel. The true leg length is the actual measurement of your legs as measured, for example, on an X-ray. The two don't always match. For example, one leg might be short, but if your pelvis and back have adapted, you might not notice because your apparent leg lengths might be the same. See chapter 8.

Who is going to be unhappier with a difference in leg length after surgery: Sally, who's had a hip fracture, or Gordon, who's been suffering from arthritis?

Sally.

In fact, Sally in general is going to be less happy. Sally had absolutely no pain before her fracture. She wants to be good as new after the surgery. Anything less will leave her unhappy. Gordon has suffered for years. Any significant improvement should please him. So given the same result, Gordon will be more grateful.

The day before surgery why can't I eat or drink anything after midnight?

Because anesthesia relaxes the muscles around your stomach and esophagus, stomach contents can go back up toward your throat and back down into your lungs. This leads to a very serious type of pneumonia because stomach contents are very acidic and can burn through lung tissue.

If the doctor thinks I have an infection, why does he not simply prescribe antibiotics?

Antibiotics alone are often ineffective because scar tissue prevents them from reaching the infection. You'll find more details on this in chapter 18.

What can I do to prevent an infection?

Alert the doctor to the presence of drainage (liquid coming from the wound) even if the liquid appears to be no more than water. Eat well. You want a healthy mix of foods. If your appetite isn't great, consider milk shake–like products that your doctor or pharmacist can point you to.

How long should my hip or knee hurt after joint replacement surgery?

There is no specific answer to that question, because patients exhibit very different levels of pain tolerance. By and large, most of the hip pain should have resolved within a month and knee pain should be very tolerable by the end of the third month. This is a rough guideline. Patients with non-cemented ("cementless") implants may take a little longer.

Why did Sally need crutches for six weeks while Harry needed them for only four?

The two variables here are the magnitude of the surgery and the surgeon's preference. Bone is a living tissue that adapts to its surroundings. A joint replacement radically alters the forces around a hip or knee, and it will take time for the bones in those areas to adjust to this new set of forces. Excessive pressure applied to bones that are remodeling may or may not cause pain. The surgeon will combine his experience and understanding of the orthopedic literature with his knowledge of your particular operation to judge how long you should use crutches.

My hip still hurts, and my surgeon is blaming it on my back. Is he full of malarkey?

Not necessarily. It is true that hip pain can be coming from the back, even in the absence of back pain. One should be particularly suspicious of this when the hip X-rays don't suggest much pathology.

Do I need anti-rejection medications after a joint replacement?

No.

Glossary

---

acetabulum: A round depression on either side of the pelvis, it is the socket of the hip joint.

allograft: Tissue coming from someone else that will be used to compensate for deficiencies encountered during surgery. See chapter 9.

Arixtra: An injectable blood thinner. See chapters 10 and 18.

asymptomatic: Causing no symptoms.

autologous blood donation: Blood that you donate for yourself in anticipation of your surgery.

AVN (avascular necrosis): A common synonym for osteonecrosis. See Osteonecrosis.

cancellous bone: Spongy, lace-like bone (in contradistinction to cortical bone).

cement: A product used to fasten an implant to the bone. It is not sticky as it is not a glue. It works its way into the interstices of bone, much as cement does between the bricks of a wall. See chapter 8.

ceramic: A type of material used for the femoral ball or acetabular cup liner, and much more rarely for a total knee replacement. Note that there exist a number of different ceramic materials. See chapter 19.

condyle. The knob-like projection at the lower end of the femur. There are two condyles, the medial condyle on the inner part of the knee and the lateral condyle to the outside.

cortical bone: Hard, wood-like bone that forms the outer portion of all bones. Within cortical bone lies cancellous bone.

Coumadin: A time-honored pill that thins blood. See chapter 10.

CPM: An abbreviation for Continuous Passive Motion machine. This device sits on your bed and slowly bends your knee back and forth. See chapter 15.

DVT: An abbreviation for deep venous thrombosis, a potentially serious clotting in the deep veins in the thigh, calf, or pelvis. The condition can be asymptomatic (see definition above), but can also lead to leg swelling, a pulmonary embolus (see definition below), or death (needs no explanation). See chapter 18.

drop foot: A person's inability to raise the foot up. The foot droops. This results from dysfunction of the peroneal nerve, a nerve that begins in the buttock area and courses down past the knee. See chapter 18.

embolus: Traveling of an unwanted substance from one part of the body to another by way of the bloodstream. The substance usually consists of a blood clot, but can also be a fat globule or an air bubble. See Pulmonary. See chapter 18.

EMG: An abbreviation for electromyography. This is a test that evaluates the nerves and muscles by way of fine needles and an electrical current. It is prescribed in patients suspected of having dysfunction of one or more nerves. See chapter 18.

extension: Straightening of a joint.

femoral head: The ball-like protuberance at the top end of the femur. The femoral head, femoral neck, and acetabulum together form the hip joint. See chapter 7.

femoral neck: The narrow, napkin ring–like portion of the femur connecting the femoral head to the main body of the femur. See chapter 7.

femur: Thighbone. The largest bone in the body. At the top end sits the hip and at the other lies the knee. See chapter 7.

flexion: Bending of a joint.

foot drop: see Drop foot.

Fragmin: an injectable blood thinner. See chapters 10 and 18.

idiopathic: Of unknown cause.

immobilizer: A semisoft device wrapped around the leg. It provides stability to a painful or wobbly knee. It also limits the extent to which a person can bend the hip (see how far you can bend the hip when your knee is straight). See chapter 15.

knee immobilizer: See Immobilizer.

lateral: Toward the outside. The right side of a right knee is lateral.

loosening: A process by which an implant gradually becomes unattached from the surrounding bone. In some cases the implant has never been fully attached. Keep in mind that the term *loosening* is relative: The implant may not be loose to the naked eye and may be difficult to remove. See Micromotion. See chapter 18.

Lovenox: An injectable blood thinner. See chapter 10.

lucency: An x-ray finding. It is a space between the implant and the bone. It can be normal or can indicate that the implant is loose, in other words, not solidly anchored to bone. See chapter 18.

medial: Toward the midline. The left side of a right knee is medial.

micromotion: An implant can be classified as loose even if no motion is obvious. Indeed, the implant can be ever so slightly loose: not enough to be visible but enough to cause pain. See chapter 18.

osteonecrosis: This technically translates to bone death. Bone is richly supplied by blood vessels. When this circulation is interrupted, a section of bone can literally die. This is often a painful condition.

osteotomy: Surgical procedure whereby a bone is cut and its direction changed.

palsy (nerve): Dysfunction of a nerve. It can be partial or total. See chapter 18.

patella: The kneecap.

patellofemoral: Pertaining to the kneecap and the matching groove on the femur.

phlebitis: An inflammation of a vein. When it involves a superficial vein (one that is visible to the naked eye), it is usually not serious. When it concerns a deep vein, it may be associated with thrombosis, i.e., clotting, and this can pose a serious risk. See DVT.

poly: The everyday abbreviation for ultra-high molecular weight polyethylene, the "plastic" used in a joint replacement. See chapters 8 and 19.

prognosis: Anticipated outcome. Example: If the prognosis is good, you are likely to have a good outcome.

pulmonary: Pertaining to the lungs. A pulmonary embolus is a blood clot that has traveled to the lungs.

rehabilitation: "Going to rehab" means you will be receiving inpatient physical therapy, an intermediate step between hospitalization and going home.

stem (femoral): The metallic portion of the hip replacement that sits inside the femur. See Femur. See chapter 8.

stenosis: Narrowing. Spinal stenosis refers to a narrowing of the spinal canal. It can cause hip or knee pain and needs to be considered in patients exhibiting confusing symptoms. See chapter 18.

tibia: Shinbone.

trochlea. The groove at the end of the femur inside of which the kneecap glides.

type and cross (type and hold): Specimens of your blood sent to the blood bank for analysis in anticipation of your receiving a blood transfusion.

UHMWPE: The technical abbreviation for ultra-high molecular weight polyethylene, the "plastic" used in a joint replacement. See chapters 8 and 19.

valgus: An angular deformity, the apex of which points inward. Simply put, a person with valgus knees is said to be knock-kneed.

varus: The opposite of valgus. A person with varus knees is bowlegged.

Index

**OTHER TITLES FROM THE BESTSELLING SERIES
WHAT YOUR DOCTOR MAY *NOT* TELL YOU ABOUT™ . . .**

AUTOIMMUNE DISORDERS
The Revolutionary Drug-free Treatments for Thyroid
Disease · Lupus · MS · IBD · Chronic Fatigue ·
Rheumatoid Arthritis, and Other Diseases

BREAST CANCER
How Hormone Balance Can Help Save Your Life

CHILDREN'S ALLERGIES AND ASTHMA
Simple Steps to Help Stop Attacks and
Improve Your Child's Health

CHILDREN'S VACCINATIONS
Learn What You Should—and Should Not—Do to Protect
Your Kids

CIRCUMCISION
Untold Facts on America's Most Widely Performed—
and Most Unnecessary—Surgery

FIBROIDS
New Techniques and Therapies—Including
Breakthrough Alternatives

FIBROMYALGIA
The Revolutionary Treatment That Can Reverse
the Disease

FIBROMYALGIA FATIGUE
The Powerful Program That Helps
You Boost Your Energy and Reclaim Your Life

HPV AND ABNORMAL PAP SMEARS
Get the Facts on This Dangerous Virus—Protect Your
Health and Your Life!

HYPERTENSION
The Revolutionary Nutrition and Lifestyle Program to Help
Fight High Blood Pressure

HYPERTHYROIDISM
A Simple Plan for Extraordinary Results

KNEE PAIN AND SURGERY
Learn the Truth About MRIs and Common Misdiagnoses—
and Avoid Unnecessary Surgery

MENOPAUSE
The Breakthrough Book on *Natural* Hormone Balance

MIGRAINES
The Breakthrough Program That Can Help End Your Pain

OSTEOPOROSIS
Help Prevent—and Even Reverse—the Disease
That Burdens Millions of Women

PARKINSON'S DISEASE
A Holistic Program for Optimal Wellness

more . . .

PEDIATRIC FIBROMYALGIA
A Safe, New Treatment Plan for Children

PREMENOPAUSE
Balance Your Hormones and Your Life from Thirty to Fifty